Revised Edition

Bioavailability and Bioequivalence in Pharmaceutical Technology

Revised Edition

Bioavailability and Bioequivalence in Pharmaceutical Technology

Edited by

Tapan Kumar Pal

MChE (Medalist), PhD (Chem. Engg), FIE, VDI (Germany), Former DAAD Fellow (FRG)

Chief Investigator, Bioequivalence Study Centre

Professor
Department of Pharmaceutical Technology
Jadavpur University
Kolkata, West Bengal

M Ganesan

MPharm, PhD

Assistant Professor
KM College of Pharmacy
Madurai, Tamil Nadu

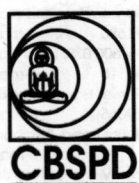

CBSPD

CBS Publishers & Distributors Pvt Ltd

New Delhi • Bengaluru • Chennai • Kochi • Kolkata • Lucknow • Mumbai
Hyderabad • Jharkhand • Nagpur • Patna • Pune • Uttarakhand

Revised Edition

**Bioavailability and
Bioequivalence in
Pharmaceutical
Technology**

ISBN: 978-81-239-1158-8

Copyright © Editors

Revised Edition: 2021
Reprint: 2023
First Edition: 2004
Reprint: 2006, 2009

Published by Satish Kumar Jain and produced by Varun Jain for
CBS Publishers & Distributors Pvt Ltd
4819/XI Prahlad Street, 24 Ansari Road, Daryaganj, New Delhi 110 002, India
Ph: 011-23289259, 23266861, 23266867   Website: www.cbspd.com
Fax: 011-23243014   e-mail: delhi@cbspd.com

Corporate Office: 204 FIE, Industrial Area, Patparganj, Delhi 110 092, India
Ph: 011-4934 4934   Fax: 011-4934 4935   e-mail: publishing@cbspd.com;
publicity@cbspd.com

Branches

- **Bengaluru:** Seema House 2975, 17th Cross, KR Road, Banasankari 2nd Stage, Bengaluru 560 070, Karnataka, India
  Ph: +91-80-26771678/79   Fax: +91-80-26771680   e-mail: bangalore@cbspd.com
- **Chennai:** 7, Subbaraya Street, Shenoy Nagar, Chennai 600 030, Tamil Nadu, India
  Ph: +91-44-26680620, 26681266   Fax: +91-44-42032115   e-mail: chennai@cbspd.com
- **Kochi:** 42/1325, 1326, Power House Road, Opp KSEB, Power House, Ernakulum Kochi 682 018, Kerala, India
  Ph: +91-484-4059061-65,67   Fax: +91-484-4059065   e-mail: kochi@cbspd.com
- **Kolkata:** 147, Hind Ceramics Compound, 1st Floor, Nilgunj Road, Belghoria, Kolkata-700056, West Bengal, India
  Ph: +033-25633055, 033-25633056   e-mail: kolkata@cbspd.com
- **Lucknow:** Basement, Khushnuma Complex, 7 Meerabai Marg (Behind Jawahar Bhawan), Lucknow-226001, UP, India
  Ph: +0522-4000032   e-mail: tiwari.lucknow@cbspd.com
- **Mumbai:** PWD Shed, Gala no 25/26, Ramchandra Bhatt Marg, Next to JJ Hospital Gate no. 2, Opp. Union Bank of India, Noorbaug, Mumbai-400009, Maharashtra, India
  Ph: 022-66661880/89   e-mail: mumbai@cbspd.com

Representatives

- Hyderabad   0-9885175004
- Patna   0-9334159340
- Jharkhand   0-9811541605
- Pune   0-9923910676
- Nagpur   0-9421945513
- Uttarakhand   0-9716462459

Printed at Glorious Printers, Jhilmil Industrial Area, Delhi, India

FOREWORD

I am happy to learn that the proceedings of the **Seminar-cum-Workshop on Bioavailability and Bioequivalence** is going to be published.

The objective of any seminar is to bring together a group of people from different fields of work and life in order to initiate a meaningful dialogue, and it is the objective of this publication to disseminate the knowledge collected there for practical use.

Bioavailability and Bioequivalence are important tools for the assessment of therapeutic efficacy of Drug. Sophisticated instrumentations involving HPLC and LC-MS and expertise are essential to carry out such study.

The purpose of this book is therefore to offer a documentation of these techniques and methodologies illustrated by experienced scientists and technologists working in this field. Moreover, the department of Pharmaceutical Technology of our University has got the approval from the Drugs Controller General of India (DCGI, Letter No. 4 14/97 DCpt(I) dt 12 Oct. 2002 to carryout Bioequivalence study.

It may also be noted that ours is the first institute in eastern region granted such approval and it is one of 12 such centres in India. Evidently this book will definitely help to accelerate the technical performance of this centre and at the same time will be useful to the large number of people engaged both in academic institutes and pharmaceutical industries who are interested in development of Bioavailability and Bioequivalence studies and research in our country.

A. N. Basu
Vice Chancellor
Jadavpur University
Kolkata 700 032

PREFACE

The patient consumes drugs (Tablets/Capsules etc.) to recover from his illness. (The function of the drug is to kill the bacteria/virus for curing the patient.) With this objective any drug should have the desired therapeutic efficacy *i.e.*, the drug should reach the blood after being absorbed with the specific concentration.

The objective of the Bioavailability study is to estimate the blood plasma concentration of the particular drug with the help of sophisticated instruments involving HPLC and to assess its therapeutic efficacy as per the guidelines of DCGI, New Delhi. Consequently the quality of the drug will be ensured for its consumption by human being. The aim of the Bioequivalence study is to compare a Test drug formulation manufactured by certain pharmaceutical company with a Standard Reference formulation of the same drug, which has been formulated by another company and is already in the market for human consumption.

As per the terms and conditions of DCGI, New Delhi it is mandatory for the pharmaceutical companies to submit the report of Bioequivalence study of new drug formulations for getting NOC from DCGI prior to its marketing although the formulations of same drug is in market with other trade name.

Moreover, based on the outcome of Bioequivalence study the pharmacokinetic parameters C_{max}, T_{max}, AUC of drug delivery systems can be evaluated. At the same time it will open up avenues of undertaking higher research in the field of drug metabolites, protein binding of drug for the improvement of therapeutic efficacy of drug.

The book illustrates the theoretical as well as practical aspects of Bioavailability & Bioequivalence study with a special emphasis on the HPLC assay procedures of some new drugs, which are not found in B.P. or U.S.P. The topic of the book is included in the curriculum of Pharmaceutical Science (B. Pharm/M. Pharm) level.

Therefore, this book will benefit the pharmacy people of academic institutes as well as the scientist and Executives of the industries who are practicing bioequivalence for their professional growth and up-gradation. Some of the books deal with the theoretical aspects of Bioavailability but this book will illustrate the in-depth technical procedure to estimate the blood plasma concentration of drug by HPLC as well as statistical evaluation of experimental data (ANOVA) in accord with the guidelines of DCGI (Drugs Controller General of India).

We would like to convey our sincere thanks to all the distinguished authors who have taken all sorts of troubles to contribute in this book.

We convey our gratitude to our respected Vice Chancellor Prof. A. N. Basu, Prof. A. R. Thakur, Pro Vice Chancellor and Prof. S. K. Sanyal, Ex-Dean, FET and Prof. R. N. Mukherjee (Ex-Professor in Chemical Engg. and my Teacher) for their continuous inspiration and encouragement.

We would like to express our sincere thanks especially to Mr. Ashis Roy, Mr. Deepnath Roychowdhury and Mr. Utpal Moitra and others of Indian Drug Manufacturers' Association (Bengal Board) for their whole hearted support and help. The financial support from All India Council of Technical Education, PEDDI and Chemito Instruments Pvt. Ltd. as well as Jadavpur University in organizing the Seminar is gratefully acknowledged.

Finally we wish to record our deep appreciation to all of our scholars and well-wishers who have come forward to make this compilation a grand success.

Prof. (Dr.) Tapan Kumar Pal
M. Ganesan

ABOUT THE CONTRIBUTORS

○ **Alekha Dash**, Ph.D. is a Professor of Pharmacy Sciences in the School of Pharmacy & Health Professions, Creighton University, Omaha, Nebraska, USA. He also serves as an Adjunct Professor, in the Department of Pharmaceutical Sciences, University of Nebraska Medical Center, College of Pharmacy. His area of teaching includes pharmaceutics, drug delivery systems, and pharmaceutical analysis. His major research focus is on pre-formulation, characterization of solid-state properties of drugs, drug delivery system design, pharmaceutical analysis and nutraceuticals. He serves in the editorial board of the Analytical Profiles Drug Substances and Excipients. He is a member of AAPS, AACP and New York Academy of Sciences. He is a consultant to many pharmaceutical and nutraceutical companies.

○ **Alok K. Ravi**, M.Sc. Ph.D. Scholar
Dr. R. P. Centre, AIIMS, New Delhi-110 029.

○ **Anil Kumar Ghosh** (b.1951), Ph.D., Bio-Chemistry - Yeast Bio-technology/Protein Chemistry/Fungal Bio-Chemistry, Recipient of Raman Research Fellowship 2000. Fellow of Indian Chemical Society and West Bengal Academy of Science and Technology. At present working at Indian Institute of Chemical Biology, 4, Raja S.C. Mullick Road, Kolkata 700032.

○ **Ms. Arjita Roy Chowdury**, MSc, HPLC Analyst, has submitted the Ph.D. thesis under the guidance of Prof. (Dr.) T. K. Pal. Presently, associated with Bioequivalence Study Centre, Jadavpur University, Kolkata. Expert in Analytical Method development, Data Interpretation, Documentation, etc.

○ **B. Sitharaman**, B.Sc. in chemistry with distinction from Madras University. Undergone the general management programme conducted by Indian Institute of Management, Ahmedabad. Written more than 50 technical write ups on various subjects on gas chromatography.
  Presently, working with Toshniwal Instruments (India) Pvt. Ltd. as Director.

O *Dipankar Malakar* (b. 1975), passed M.Sc. (Physical Chemistry) in 1999 and presently working at Indian Institute of Chemical Biology, 4 Raja S. C. Mullick Road, Kolkata-700032, as a project assistant in a project namely "Bio-efficacy and analytical evaluation of herbal active molecules" under the supervision of Dr. A. K. Ghosh.

O *Mr. H. Roustai*, is currently a fourth year Pharm. D. student in the School of Pharmacy and Health Professions, Creighton University, Omaha, Nebraska, USA.

O *Prof. Krishnangshu Ray*, MBBS, MD, PhD, DA, FACCP. Presently Professor of Pharmacology, NRS Medical College, Kolkata as well as Director, Drugs Control, Govt. of West Bengal. Prof. Ray has got 20 years of teaching experience in various Universities in India and abroad. He is the recipient of WHO fellowship and International Fellowship in Medical Education in UK, USA and Karolinska Institute, Sweden.
His fields of interest are Clinical Pharmacology and Medical Ethics.

O *Ms. Mausumi Chakravarthi*, MSc, HPLC Analyst, has submitted the Ph.D. thesis under the guidance of Prof. (Dr.) T. K. Pal. Presently, associated with Bioequivalence Study Centre, Jadavpur University, Kolkata. Expert in Analytical Method Development, Data Interpretation, Documentation, etc.

O *Mr. M. Jayakumar*, M. Pharm, HPLC Analyst. Presently working as Senior Research Fellow in the DST (New Delhi) funded project entitled "Development of Controlled Release Contraceptive Device containing Hormones." He has shown his active involvement in analytical method development, Clinical Studies, etc. at Bioequivalence Study Centre, Jadavpur University, Kolkata.

O *Nageshwar Rao Thudi*, B. Pharm., Worked as Scientist in clinical research in Vimta Labs Ltd., Hyderabad, Andhra Pradesh during 1999 to 2003. Presently associated as Research Scientist - Clinical Development, Chembiotek Research International, Plot No. 7, Sector V, Salt Lake, Kolkata-700064.

O *Nilima Biswas* (b.1966), Ph.D., Biochemistry/Enzymology/ Molecular Biology/Virology. Member of the American Society of Microbiology. At present at University of California, San Diego. 9500 Gilman Drive. La Jolla, CA 92093-0366.

○ *Dr. N. R. Biswas*, M.D., DM, DNB, DSc., Addl. Professor of Ocular Pharmacology, Dr. R.P. Centre, AIIMS, New Delhi-110023. He is having 14 years of teaching experience and publication more than 100 papers in reputed National and International Journals.

○ *Prof. (Dr.) S. Bhattacharyya*, M.B.B.S., M.D. (Pharmacology), FAMS, He is Ex-Professor and Head, Department of Pharmacology, Institute of Medical Science, Banaras Hindu University. His last assignment was as Emeritus Scientist in Indian Council of Medical Research, New Delhi.

He had 38 years experience in teaching & research, and around 400 publications. The editors deeply regret Dr. Bhattacharyya's sudden demise in 2003.

○ *Prof. (Dr.) S. K. Garg*, M.Pharm., Ph.D., Professor & more than 35 years teaching and research experience in the department of Pharmacology, Post-graduate Institute of Medical Education and Research, Chandigarh-160012 (India).

○ *Prof. S. N. Banerjee*, MBBS, MD, FCCP. Primarily Professor of Pharmacology, West Bengal Medical Education Service and presently he is the Special Secretary, Medical Education, Govt. of West Bengal. Prof. Banerjee held the prestigious administrative positions of Principal Medical College and Calcutta National Medical College, Kolkata. He posses 30 years of teaching and research experience.

○ *Subhabrata Sengupta*, D.Sc., is working in the field of microbial biotechnology for the last 30 years. His major contributions are in the fields of peptide antibiotics, amino acid fermentations and hydrogen biotechnology. He extensively studied a huge numbers of commercial glycosidase enzymes of higher fungi and indicated their applications in bioprocess development. He has 84 research publications and 8 national and international patents. He is now Director Grade Scientist in Indian Institute of Chemical Biology (CSIR), Calcutta.

○ *Mr. Subhabrata Dey*, M.Sc. He is working as in charge of HPLC unit, Department of CRIF, Chittaranjan National Cancer Institute, Kolkata. He completed upgraded training course on HPLC at USA and honored as visiting lecturer at different Universities of the country for the last few years. He is working exhaustively on the application of this challenging technology in the field of pharmaceutics.

○ *Dr. T. K. Chattaraj*, MBBS, MD (Pharmacology) Associate Professor, NRS Medical College, Kolkata. Also he is been associated with Bioequivalence Study Centre, Jadavpur University, Kolkata as Clinical Pharmacologist. He's been always interested in the fields like Clinical Pharmacokinetics, Ethical Issues, etc.

○ *Dr. T. C. Chawla*, M.Sc., Ph.D., Scientist-II, Dr. R. P. Centre, AIIMS, New Delhi-110029 having 12 years of teaching experience published 30 papers in National and International Journals.

○ *Mr. U. Mandal*, B. Pharm, Presently doing his M. Pharm and working with the Bioequivalence projects. He has been actively engaged in Method Development, Data Interpretation, etc. in the Bioequivalence Study Centre, Jadavpur University, Kolkata.

○ *Dr. Vandana Dixit* is the Director of Anal Chem Pvt. Ltd. (only manufacturer of Solid Phase Extraction products in India). She received her Ph.D. degree from University of Utah, Salt Lake City, USA in organic chemistry and was Production and Quality Manager in Varian Sample Preparation Products, USA for several years.

○ *Dr. Vivek R. Dhole*, M.Sc , Ph.D. He has been awarded Govt. of India's, Home Minister Award as the Best Scientist in the year 1998 for the research contribution in the fields of petroleum fuel and petrochemicals analysis. He has published more than 40 papers in the national and international journals and conferences. Previously worked as Asst. Director and Head of the Analytical and Instrumentation Division of Forensic Science Laboratory, Govt. of Maharashtra, at Mumbai, Nagpur and Pune. Presently working with Toshniwal/Chemito Instruments Pvt. Ltd., as the Sr. Manager.

○ *Dr. Vyas M. Dixit*, is the Managing Director of Anal Chem Pvt. Ltd. He received his Ph.D. degree from CDRI, Lucknow. He was Faculty Intern at University of Utah in the Chemistry Department. He also worked at Varian Sample Preparation Products as Research and Development Manager for several years.

CONTENTS

ETHICAL ISSUES INVOLVED IN BIOEQUIVALENCE STUDY

Dr. Krishnangshu Ray*
Prof. (Dr.) Soumendra Nath Banerjee**

'The health of my patient will be my first consideration and a physician shall act only in the patient's interest when providing medical care which might have the effect of weakening the physical and mental condition of the patient'

World Medical Association

PRELUDE

Ethics is defined as reasoned analysis of human duty. In the context of clinical research ethics could be of two types: (*a*) individual ethics which refers to duty of an experimenter to apply existing knowledge for the best possible treatment for every subject and (*b*) collective ethics that relates to the duty of the experimenter to acquire new knowledge so that such advances benefit future subjects and having acquired new knowledge, to communicate it accurately with other experimenters. During drug development research ethical issues are relevant irrespective of the quality whether it is therapeutic (patient study) or non-therapeutic (volunteer study). There should not remain any conflict of interests between a doctor's role as a therapist and as a drug developer. Only difference is that the Clinical Trials are better structured, better organized and enables conclusive about the value of therapy to be drawn with greater certainty and speed. The 'Nuremberg Code' of biomedical ethics was the first eye-opener by convicting 18 out of 25 medical personnel found guilty of war crimes against involuntary human subjects. In 1964 World Medical Association formulated the 'Helsinki Declaration' addressing the ethical, moral and legal issues of human experimentation. Later, it was amended in 1975 at Venice, Italy. The latest modification took place at the WMA General Assembly held at Edinburgh, Scotland. However, Indian Council of Medical research (ICMR) in 1980 issued a similar guideline

*Professor of Pharmacology, NRS Medical College, Kolkata.
**Principal, Medical College, Kolkata.

in accordance with the law and regulations of the country ensuring a better protection for the subjects.

BASIC PRINCIPLES OF MEDICAL ETHICS IN HUMAN RESEARCH

(a) Principle of *Justice* that fairly distributes the benefits and burdens of the research. Research participants assume some risk in order to benefit society as a whole. Therefore, no single group, especially not disadvantaged, vulnerable or minority groups, should be asked to bear a disproportionate share of the risk.

(b) Principle of *Respect for persons* requiring investigators to treat subjects as autonomous individuals and obtain Informed Consents before participating the research. Research subjects must not be regarded as passive sources of data, but as individuals whose welfare and rights must be respected. Treating them as partners or collaborators improve the quality of research and compliance.

(c) Principle of *Beneficience* that requires investigators to design protocol that provide valid and generalized knowledge and to ensure that the benefits of the research are proportionate to the risks assumed by the subjects. The researcher must try to minimize the risks and maximize the benefits of the participants.

Ethical Considerations During Human Experimentation

(a) Risks of subjects are minimized and proportionate to the anticipated benefits and knowledge

(b) Data are monitored to ensure safety of the subjects

(c) Selection of subjects is equitable

(d) Additional safeguards to be adopted in case of vulnerable subjects

(e) Informed consents to be obtained if appropriate

(f) Confidentiality and privacy to be adequately ensured.

Ethical Exemptions During Human Experimentation

(a) Surveys or interviews except in cases of liability, financial loss, reduced employability, research upon drug abuse etc.

(b) Observation of public behaviour

(c) Research on normal educational practices

(d) Studies on existing records, data, diagnostic or pathological specimens provided that the data can not be linked to individual subject.

BIOEQUIVALENCE STUDY: AN ETHICAL UNDERTAKING

Bioequivalence refer to the comparison of bioavailabilities of different formulations, drug products or batches of the same drug product. The availability to the biological system of a drug or chemical substance formulated into a pharmaceutical product is integral to the goals of dosage from design and paramount to the effectiveness of the medication. Any generic drug product is considered bioequivalent to the brand drug product if its rate and extent of systemic absorption do not have therapeutically significant difference when administered at the same dose of the active ingredient of same chemical form, in similar dosage form, by the same route of administration under the same experimental conditions. Bioequivalence studies are necessary during the selection of drug products for any given population since:

(*a*) the generic substitution of drug is the process of dispensing different brand or unbranded drug in the place of prescribed drug product. The substituted product must be therapeutically equivalent to the prescribed product so that it produces similar therapeutic response

(*b*) the therapeutic substitution of a drug is the process of dispensing a therapeutic alternative in place of the prescribed drug product *e.g.* amoxycillin is dispensed for penicillin

(*c*) the preparation of a Drug Formulary for any hospital or health institute to provide drug information and guidelines for rational use of drugs

(*d*) to obtain the FDA approval for determining its prescribability

(*e*) individual bioequivalence study is required to identify the individual variability which is essential for the switchability of a drug.

INFORMED CONSENTS: AN ETHICAL DOCUMENT

Written consent forms are required to document the discussions between the investigator and the volunteer. The form should be duly signed by both the parties and must be structured by avoiding technical jargon and complicated sentences that are incomprehensible to lay persons. Simple, clear and preferably local language to be used regarding the disclosure process and sufficient time has to the permitted to each subject for making thoughtful decisions about participation. 'Surrogate Consents' or 'Power of Attorney' must be enforced in case of mentally ill or incapacitated subjects. Every volunteer must receive the following information before participating in Bioequivalence study:

(*a*) the nature of the research project by explicit description about the purpose of the study, names with affiliations of the investigator and process of recruitment of subjects (*n*) the procedures of the study which involves the nature of sampling, design and duration of the study with detail of standard care that is to be undertaken during the study protocol

(*c*) assurances regarding the voluntariness in participation and withdrawal from the project at any time

(*d*) potential risks and hazards while conducting the study including medical, psychological, social and economic harms and benefits as well as its measures of protection should be clearly explained

(*e*) openness of the investigator regarding any queries as well as the confidentiality of the study must be enforced to the participants. In case of the bioequivalence study of anti-HIV drugs the value of privacy is enormous since threatening of it might stigmatize the volunteer in his/her employment, society or insurance.

SELECTION OF SUBJECTS FOR BIOEQUIVALENCE STUDY

Irrespective of 'single dose' or 'multiple dose' bioequivalence studies, each volunteer should be healthy, age ranging between 18-55 years, preferably males (females of child bearing age group are usually exempted), non-smoker, non-alcoholic, normal body weight according to accepted life tables. Preliminary screening for the suitability by means of extensive medical history, clinical and laboratory values must be obtained. Depending upon the therapeutic class and the safety profile of the drug special investigations may have to be carried out beforehand. Standardization of diet, fluid intake, exercise, posture, concomitant drug administration must be performed. Any beverage or diet containing alcohol or fruit juices containing xanthine compounds likely to affect the hepatic and renal functions should be restricted during the study period. Sometimes patients instead of healthy volunteers may have to be incorporated in bioequivalence study specially when the investigational compound is known to have adverse potential to be considered unacceptable for healthy individuals. Phenotyping and/or genotyping of subjects may be considered for safety or pharmacokinetic reasons.

CLINICAL PHARMACOLOGIST: THE CUSTODIAN OF ETHICS

Clinical Pharmacologist being the member of the study group should be scientifically competent to design protocols in an objective and rigorous manner. He/she should promote appropriate attention to the ethical issues in professional meetings and publications in their institutions and in their specific projects. Conscientious and ethically sensitive investigators are always ideal. An investigator must realize that the different roles they play may create the 'conflicts of interests'. A clinical pharmacologist who is also a personal physician for his/her study subjects must appreciate what is best for the research project. In such conditions he/she is in dilemma whether to enroll or to remain on a standardized protocol rather than individualizing care when problems arise. Again, fraudulence in biomedical research like fabrication of data is another blatant example of unethical research practice. In many cases, the clinical investigator for financial interest misinform or disinform study subjects which may be stamped as 'deception in research'.

INSTITUTIONAL REVIEW BOARD (ETHICAL COMMITTEE)

Ethical Committee ensures that the research is ethically acceptable, welfare and rights of the volunteers are protected. The Committee should be decentralized and typically consists of researchers, clinical staff, patient advocates, lay members or consumers and persons knowledgeable about legal and ethical issues concerning research. The Committee places more emphasis on consent forms and on other ethical issues. The limitation of this body is its inability to monitor whether the research was actually undertaken in accordance with the submitted protocol that was approved. Investigator and sponsor have binding to inform the Ethical Committee if there is any deviation from the approved protocol.

The submitted protocol must specify the analytical procedures in detail. It should also specify the methods of handling the drop-outs and for identifying implausible outliers. Post-hoc exclusion of outliers is not generally accepted. If modeling assumption made in the protocol (*e.g.* for extrapolating AUC to infinity) turn out to be invalid, a revised analysis in addition to the planned analysis (if feasible) should be presented and discussed.

RATIONAL APPROACHES TOWARDS SAMPLE BIOANALYSIS

The bioanalytical methods used to determine the active principle and/or its biotransformation products in plasma, serum, urine or any other suitable matrix must be well characterized, validated and documented to yield reliable results that can be satisfactorily interpreted. The main objective of validation method is to demonstrate the reliability of a particular method for the quantitative determination of an analyte's concentration in a specific matrix. Reliability of the analytical results depends upon: (*i*) *Stability* of the analytes in the biological matrix under processing conditions and during the entire period of storage (*ii*) *Specificity* (*iii*) *Accuracy* (*iv*) *Sensitivity* (*v*) *Precision* (*vi*) *Response Function*.

The validation of a bioanalytical method should comprise of two distinct phases: (*i*) the pre-study phase in which the assay is developed to comply with the six characteristics listed above and (*ii*) the study phase itself in which the validated bioanalytical method is applied to the actual analysis of samples from biostudy mainly evaluating stability, accuracy and reproducibility. All procedures should be performed according to pre-established Standard Operating Procedures (SOPs). All relevant procedures and formulate used to validate the bioanalytical method should be submitted and discussed. Any modification of the bioanalytical method before and during analysis of study specimens requires revalidation.

The test product used in the bioequivalence study must be prepared in accordance with GMP (Good Manufacturing Practice) guidelines. This should be manufactured by such process which meaningfully simulates that which will be used in production.

DATA ANALYSIS AND STATISTICS

The primary concern in bioequivalence assessment is to limit the risk of erroneously accepting bioequivalence which should not exceed the normal risk of 5% and to try to minimize the risk of erroneously rejecting bioequivalence. The statistical method for testing bioequivalence is based upon the 90% confidence interval for the ratio of the population means for the parameters under consideration. This method is equivalent to the corresponding two one-sided test procedure with the Null hypothesis of bioequivalence at the 5% significance level. The statistical analysis ANOVA (Analysis of Variance) should take into account source of variation that can be reasonably assumed to have an effect on the response. The validity of the assumptions underlying the statistical analysis (*e.g.* additivity, normality) may often be improved by transforming the raw data prior to analysis, preferably using a logarithmic transformation.

SUMMARY

The bioequivalence study involving human subjects must obey the following ethical and legal guidelines: (*i*) the risks to subjects should be minimum and be proportionate to the anticipated benefits and knowledge (*ii*) the selection of subjects should be equitable (*iii*) if subjects are vulnerable, additional safeguards to be provided (*iv*) consents should be obtained from the subjects following proper information and not merely the signature (*v*) participation of the subjects should be voluntary (*vi*) the results should be confidential (*vii*) provision of continuing opportunity to answer questions should be available (*viii*) institutional review board must review the protocol to ensure that it complies with above criteria (*ix*) investigators must develop for the task of assuring that their research is ethical. It is concluded that the interest of the science should never take precedence over considerations related to the well-being of the volunteer.

REFERENCES

Levine, R. J. (1986). *Ethics and Regulation of Clinical Research.* Baltimore. Urban and Schwarzenberg.

Veatch, R. M. (1987). *The Patient as Partner: A Theory of Human Experimentation Ethics.* Bloomington. Indian University Press.

Holder, Ar. (1985). When researchers are served subpoenas. *IRB,* **7**: 5-7.

Shapiro, M. F. and Charrow, R. P. (1985). Scientific misconduct in investigational drug trials. *N. Eng. J. Med.,* **312**: 731-736.

Kopelman, L. (1983). Randomized clinical trials: Consent and the therapeutic relationship. *Clin Res,* **31**: 1-11.

Annas, G. I., Glantz, L. H. (1986). Rules for research in nursing homes. *N. Eng. J. Med.,* **315**: 1157-1158.

Bayer, R., Levine, C. and Murray, T. H. (1984). Guidelines for confidentiality in research in AIDS. *IRB,* **6**: 1-7.

American Psychological Association (1982) Ethical Principles in the Conduct of Research with Human Participants. Washington DC, American Psychological Association.

Ellenberg, S. S. (1984). Randomization Designs in Comparative Clinical Trial. *N. Eng. J. Med.,* **310**: 1404-1408.

Angell, M. (1984). Patient preferences in randomized clinical trials. *N. Eng. J. Med.,* **310**: 1385-1387.

Endrenyi, L. (1994). A method for the evaluation of individual bioequivalence. *Int. J. Clin. Pharmacol Ther.,* **32**: 497-508.

Liu, J. P. and Weng, C. S. (1991). Detection of outlying data in bioavailability/bioequivalence studies. *Stat. Med.,* **10**: 1357-1389.

Lund, R. E. (1975). Tables for an approximate test outliers in linear models. *Technometric,* **17**: 473-476.

Holder, A. R. (1982). Do researchers and subjects have a fiduciary relationship? *IRB,* **4**: 6-7.

2

UNDERSTANDING BIOAVAILABILITY

CH. V. Rao*, B. Mishra* and S. K. Bhattacharyya*

INTRODUCTION

Bioavailability describes the amount of active drug given in a pharmacological dose, which reaches the systemic circulation after oral administration. Till fairly recently, it was assumed that all formulations, containing similar quantities of a particular drug, had the same bioavailability and were, therefore, therapeutically equivalent. Unfortunately, this assumption is not always true and it has become apparent that different formulations of the same drug are not therapeutically equivalent as their bioavailability differs. Thus, it is now important for the clinician to understand and appreciate the principles underlying the concept of bioavailability and its practical applications.

The bioavailability of a drug is more strictly defined as the amount and the rate at which the orally administered drug reaches the biological system in an active form, capable of exerting the desired pharmacological effect, including its onset, intensity and duration of action.

The bioavailability or systemic availability of an orally administered drug depends largely on the absorption and the extent of hepatic metabolism on its first-pass through the liver in addition to its action at the level of the receptors. In practice, bioavailability is determined by assessing its plasma or urine concentration over a given time following oral administration. To be therapeutically equivalent, different formulations of the same drug have to be bioequivalent, implying that they must have a similar systemic availability. Many studies have indicated that products from different manufacturers, and even different batches of drugs from the same pharmaceutical house, are not bioequivalent and have dissimilar systemic availability. While major differences in bioavailability are likely to be of clinical relevance, small differences are also important in those drugs which have a steep dose-response curve or a narrow margin of safety. Fortunately most drugs have relatively flat dose-response curves, so that only marked

*Department of Pharmacology and Pharmaceutics, Institute of Medical Sciences, Banaras Hindu University, Varanasi, U.P.

differences in bioequivalence will produce difference in therapeutic equivalence.

The currently available compendial standards laid down for bio-equivalence, including the testing of the finished product or the specifications for the raw materials and manufacturing process, leave much to be desired. The problem is particularly acute in India where such specifications either do not exist or are largely ignored, since bioavailability studies are rarely done or compared with acceptable standards which meet compendial criteria. While bioequivalence studies are not absolute guarantee of therapeutic equivalence for all drugs they ensure and are recognized to be the only certain criteria for product equivalence. The practical relevance of bio-availability was highlighted by the dramatic increase in the adverse effects of phenytoin in Australia during 1968-69. The cause was finally traced to the fact that a change in the excipient of phenytoin capsules led to a marked increase in the absorption of the drug and a consequent increase in its toxicity. Bioequivalence problems with phenytoin manufactured by different pharmaceutical concerns are also on record. In 1969, 15 of the 16 oxytetracycline brands available in the USA were discontinued because they did not meet the standard bioavailability specifications. Bioinequivalence has been reported for several other drugs including digoxin, quinidine, nalidixic acid, atenolol, propranolol, several antibiotics and non-steroidal anti-inflammatory agents. This list is likely to be far more extensive in India and can lead to widely different clinical responses to important and life-saving drugs. It is, therefore, important that the prescriber always poses the question will the drug get to its site of action in optimal therapeutic concentrations?

ASSESSMENT OF BIOAVAILABILITY

For assessing the bioavailability or clinical availability of a drug, its rate and extent of absorption and its first-pass metabolism must be evaluated. Ideally, the clinical response of the patient or the amount of the active drug at the target site of action at different time periods following administration of the drug formulation, should be assessed. However, these criteria are difficult, or even impossible, to quantify. Hence, the methods used to assess bioavailability depend upon the assumption that measurement of the drug concentration in a suitable body fluid, such as blood, plasma, serum, urine or sometime saliva, over a period of time following extra vascular administration can be correlated with its clinical availability and, therefore, with the clinical efficacy of the drug in a given disease.

Bioavailability is usually determined by the following methods:

1. Determination of whole blood, plasma or serum concentrations of the unchanged drug, either after single dose administration or in a

dosage interval at the steady state after multiple dose administration
(Figs. 1 and 2).

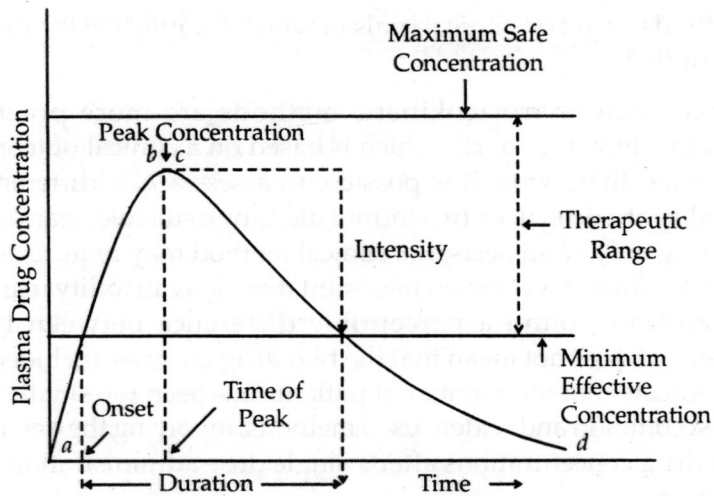

Fig. 1: Plasma Cocentration-Time Curve Followig a Single Oral Dose Showing
Bioavailability and Pharmacological Parameters
a-b: Absorption phase of curve
c-d: Elimination phase of curve

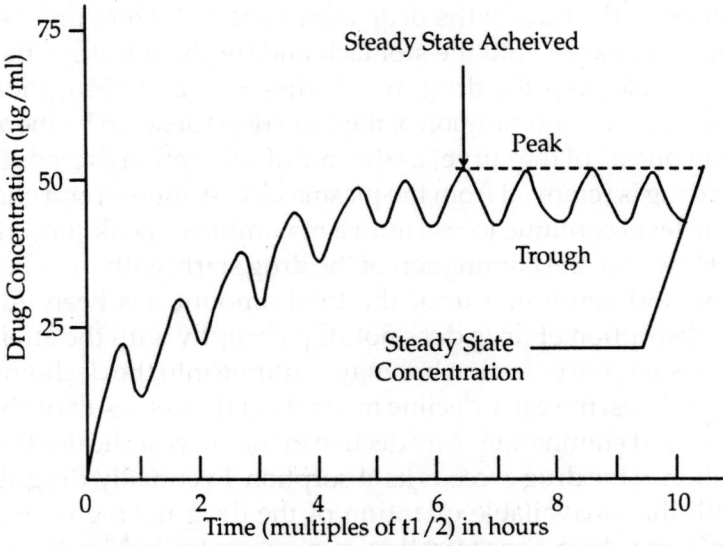

Fig. 2: Plasma Concentration Profile of a Drug Given at Half-life Intervals

2. Determination of the total amount of unchanged drug excreted in the
   urine either after single dose administration or after multiple dose
   administration in the steady state.

3. Determination of the total amount of a major metabolite of the drug excreted in the urine either after a single dose or at the steady state after multiple dose administration.

4. Methods based on clinical trials in which the effect of the drug can be quantified.

The first three pharmacokinetic methods are more practical and discriminative than the fourth which is based on a clinical outcome. It has been estimated that, while it is possible to assess a 25% difference in the bioavailability of a drug from two formulations by a suitable pharmacokinetic method using only 12 subjects, the clinical method may require as many as 1000 subjects. Thus, if a clinician has estimated bioavailability using, say, 50 patients and not found a perceptible difference between two drug formulations, it does not mean that the two drug dosages are bioequivalent but may indicate that the number of patients has been too small.

The most common and widely used methods, involving the determination of plasma drug concentrations after a single dose administration of a drug are as follows:

PLASMA CONCENTRATION–TIME CURVES

A typical plasma concentration-time curve, following a single oral dose administration of a drug formulation is depicted in Fig. 1. The plasma drug concentration at the time of the drug administration (zero time) should be nil. As the drug passes into the stomach and/or the intestine, the product disintegrates releasing the drug, which dissolves and absorption ensues. Initially the plasma concentration of the drug rises (denoted by the ascending 'absorption phase' of the curve) as the rate of absorption exceeds the rate at which the drug is removed from the plasma by distribution and elimination. The plasma level continue to rise until a maximum or peak concentration is attained. However, the elimination of the drug starts with its appearance in the plasma and continued until the total amount has been eliminated. Similarly, absorption of drug does not stop abruptly with the attainment of the peak plasma concentration but may continue into the declining portion of the curve. Thus, the early decline may reflect the net result of absorption, distribution and elimination. Any decline in the curve indicates that the rate of elimination of the drug exceeds its absorption. Eventually, drug absorption ceases with the bioavailable quantum of the drug having been absorbed and the plasma drug concentration is now controlled by the rate of its elimination by metabolism and/or excretion (elimination phase of the curve). Thus drug distribution to the tissues and extracellular fluid, as well as absorption and elimination, will affect the shape of the plasma concentration-time curve (Fig. 1).

Based on the plasma concentration-time curve, the following measurements important for bioavailability studies can be assessed (Fig. 1).

Peak concentration (C_{max}) represents the highest concentration attained by the drug in the plasma. At this concentration (point), rate of drug input becomes equal to rate of drug output.

Time of peak concentration (T_{max}) is the time required to achieve the peak plasma concentration after single dose administration of the drug, and can be used to assess the rate of absorption.

Minimum effective plasma concentration: The minimum plasma concentration of the drug required to achieve a given pharmacological or therapeutic response. This value varies from drug to drug and from individual to individual as well as with the type and severity of the disease.

Maximum safe concentration: The plasma concentration of the drug beyond which adverse effects are likely to occur.

Therapeutic range: The range of plasma drug concentrations in which the desired response is achieved yet avoiding adverse effects. The aim in clinical practice is to maintain plasma drug concentration within the therapeutic range.

Onset of action is the time required to achieve the minimum effective plasma concentration following administration of the drug formulation.

Duration of action of the therapeutic effect of the drug is defined as the time period during which the plasma concentration of the drug exceeds the minimum effective level.

Intensity of action: In general, the difference between the peak plasma concentration and the minimum effective plasma concentration provides a relative measure of the intensity of the therapeutic response of the drug.

Total area under the curve (AUC) is related to the total amount of the drug absorbed into the systemic circulation following the administration of a single dose of the formulation. However, changes in AUC may not necessarily reflect changes in the total amount of drug absorbed, but the modifications in the kinetics distribution, metabolism and excretion of the drug as well. AUC can be measured mathematically by using a technique known as the trapezoidal rule.

A hypothetical example can explain how differences in bioavailability of a given drug from different formulations marketed by various firms, can result in a patient being either over-, under- or correctly-medicated. Single equal doses of four different products of the same drug, *A*, *B*, *C* and *D*, were orally administered to the same healthy individual on four separate occasion. The plasma drug concentration-time curves were assessed (Fig. 3). If it is assumed that all the other factors with the exception of the formulation factor are the same in each case, then it is reasonable to conclude that the differences in the four curves are solely due to differences in the rate and extent of absorption of the drug from each formulation. However, each formulation (Fig. 3) results in different peak plasma concentrations (C_{max}). The AUC for products *A* and *B* are almost similar, indicating that the drug is absorbed to a similar extent from these formulations. However, the T_{max} indicates that the drug is absorbed faster from product *A* than from products *B* or *C*. Thus product *A* will act more quickly but is likely to result in adverse effects since its C_{max} exceeds the maximum safe concentration. On the other hand, product B which has a slower onset of action because it is absorbed slowly, is less likely to induce adverse effects since its C_{max} lies within the therapeutic range. Furthermore, this product has a longer duration of action than product *A*. These attributes may make product *A* more useful clinically than product *A*. Product *C* has a much smaller AUC, indicating that only a fraction of the administered does has been absorbed. In addition, this product is also absorbed slowly, as shown by its longer T_{max}, and thus does not reach the minimum effective clinically, if given as a single dose. Product *D* though exhibits lower peak drug level than product *A* and *B* and similar rate of drug absorption to that of product *A* and *B* and similar rate of drug absorption to that of product *B* (T_{max} of *B* and *D* are equal), *D* is clinically more beneficial as it maintained the drug concentration in therapeutic range for much longer period of time, *i.e.*, duration of action provided by product *D* is approximately two time more than product *A* and *B*. Product *D* is more desirable form of a dosage form specially for drugs with narrow safety margin and relatively shorter half life.

Absolute bioavailability of a drug in a formulation administered by an extravascular, including the oral route reaching the systemic circulation is the fraction of the same dose of the drug administered intavenously. In the latter case the entire administered drug dose is directly introduced into the systemic circulation and is, therefore, considered to be totally (100%) bioavailable, whereas in the former instance the drug has to be absorbed to reach the systemic circulation. Absolute bioavailability can be calculated from the formula:

$$\text{Absolute bioavailability} = \frac{(AUC)abs}{(AUC)iv}$$

where (AUC)abs and (AUC)iv are the total areas under the curve following administration of a single dose of the drug via a given absorption site and by rapid intravenous injection, respectively.

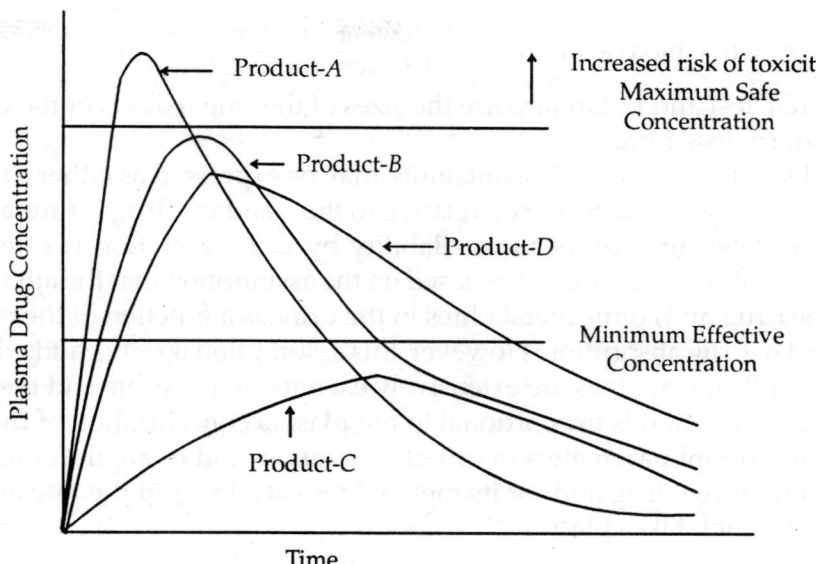

Fig. 3: Plasma Concentration-Time Curves Following Single Oral Dose of Four Formulation of the Same Drug

The above formula holds true when the same doses are used for both routes. However, when these doses are different, a correction for the dose size is made:

$$\text{Absolute bioavailability} = \frac{(AUC)abs \times Div}{(AUC)iv \times Dabs}$$

where Dabs is the size of the single dose administered via the absorption site and Div is the dose size administered intravenously.

Relative bioavailability is a measure of the fraction of a given drug that is absorbed into the systemic circulation from a particular dose compared to a clinically proven standard dose of the same drug. This is determined when a particular drug cannot be administered in the form of an intravenous bolus injection. The test dose and the standard dose, containing equal amounts of the drug, are administered via the same route to the same individual on different occasions, and the calculation is done on the basis of the plasma concentration time curves:

$$\text{Relative bioavailability} = \frac{(AUC)test}{(AUC)standard}$$

where (AUC)test and (AUC)standard are the total areas under the curve following administration of a single test dose and the standard dose.

However, when different test and standard doses are administered, a correction is made for the size of the dose:

$$\text{Relative bioavailability} = \frac{(AUC)\text{test} \times D \text{ standard}}{(AUC)\text{standard} \times D\text{test}}$$

where Dtest and Dstandard are the sizes of the single doses of the test and standard dose forms.

Absolute or relative bioavailability may be expressed as either a fraction or percentage of the test drug relative to the standard drug formulation.

The determination of bioavailability by urine excretion is often used because of convenience and is based on the assumption that the appearance of the drug and/or its metabolites in the urine is a function of the rate and extent of drug absorption. However, this assumption is only valid when the drug or its metabolites are extensively excreted in the urine and the rate of urinary excretion is proportional to the plasma concentration of the drug. The important parameters in urinary excretion studies are the cumulative amount of the drug and/or its metabolites excreted and the rate at which this excretion takes place.

FACTORS AFFECTING BIOAVAILABILITY

A wide range of factors can influence the bioavailability of a drug, the detailed discussion of which is beyond the scope of this article. Basically, the availability of the drug or its active metabolite (when a pro-drug is rendered pharmacologically active following biotransformation by metabolic processes) to the target organ or receptor is controlled by three principal factors:

1. The rate and extent of drug release from its formulation, and its subsequent absorption.
2. The first-pass effect while passing through the liver after absorption.
3. The conjoint effect of plasma protein binding, drug distribution to various body fluids, metabolism and excretion.

The factors which influence bioavailability are:

Physiological factors: These include the effect of gastrointestinal fluids (pH, mucus, bile salts, complexing components); motility (gastric emptying, presence of food, rest and exercise); gastrointestinal transit time (which can be affected by a large number of drugs); absorption surface (physiological integrity, area and blood flow); metabolism of drugs by the gut wall, liver, skin and bronchial mucosa; the pharmacogenetic factors determining the rate of hepatic metabolism; disease states such as malabsorption, achlorhydria, throtoxicosis and coeliac disease; the gut flora and the age, sex, weight and physical status of the patient and the route of administration.

Physico-chemical factors: These include the drugs' lipid and water solubility, partition coefficient, dissociation constant, polymorphic form, surface area, particle size, crystal shape, stability, biophysical factors related to the absorptive membrane, the solvent and the effect of its complexing agent.

Pharmacological factors: These are outlined in Table 1.

The bioavailability of a drug given chronically may differs from that given in a single dose, since the metabolism of the drug at the first-pass can be saturated by the gut and hepatic enzymes.

TABLE 1: PHARMACOLOGICAL FACTORS AFFECTING BIOAVAILABILITY

Factor	Possible Cause/Effect
Variation in drug content	Inadequate quality control
Storage (drug and excipient stability)	Loss of effect (nitroglycerine)
State of drug	
Particle size	Variable effect (anticoagulants)
Polymorphism	Different crystalline forms differ in dissolution rate (steroids, barbiturates)
Solvate/hydrate*	Variable bioavailability (ampicilin)
Salts	Dissolution rate with sodium salts better (sodium tolbutamide)
Esters	Antibiotic esters have increased bio-availability
pH	
Excipients	Dilantin mixed with calcium sulphate increases toxicity

*Solvate when a molecule of solvent enters the crystal structure. If the solvent is water it is known as a hydrate.

Saturation Kinetics: Most drugs are subject to first order kinetics, where the rate of metabolism is directly proportional to the drug concentration. However, the hepatic metabolic capacity for some drugs can become saturated, leading to zero order kinetics where the unmetabolized drug remains in the circulation since the rate of metabolism is now constant and independent of the amount of the drug present. This phenomenon may explain the sudden unexpected toxicity of drugs such as phenytoin, theophylline or ethanol, since when saturation occurs a moderate increase in the dose may produce a disproportionately large increase in the circulating concentration of the unmetabolized active drug. Saturation kinetics also explain the accumulation of drugs undergoing substantial first-pass metabolism during chronic dosing, which results in saturation of the hepatic microsomal enzymes responsible for drug metabolism.

CONCLUSION

An understanding of the bioequivalence of different drug products is a prerequisite for predicting their therapeutic equivalence. Drugs with a narrow therapeutic range and dose-dependent kinetics require greater attention as they are likely to have a high-risk potential. Even small changes in the bioavailability profile of such drugs can cause major changes in the plasma drug concentration and consequent toxicity. The therapeutic efficacy and safety to many drugs commonly used in clinical practice can be augmented by individualization of their dosage. Administration of the 'usual' or 'average' doses can be considered satisfactory only when the therapeutic margin of the drug is so large that such doses can be efficacious in the majority of patients and excessive only in a minority. This holds true for only a fraction of the clinically useful drugs. With the other drugs, unless their dosage is adjusted to the clinical needs and tolerance of an individual patient, they are likely to be ineffective in some patients and induce serious adverse effects in others.

Drug manufacturing in this country has been reduced to the level of a cottage industry, with little or no effective quality control measures being exercised by appropriate drug control authorities. It is, therefore, not surprising that different drug formulations of the same drug, marketed by different pharmaceutical firms, have widely differing bioavailability profiles. Special caution has to be exercised with the 'fast release' and 'slow release' formulations. It is likely that the former will overshoot the maximum safe concentrations and induce adverse effects, while the latter may not achieve the minimum effective concentrations. In addition, patients accustomed to a fast release formulation may not achieve therapeutic levels of the drug when a change is made to a slow release preparation. Similarly, if patients are accustomed to a slow release formulation, higher, and possibly toxic levels of the drug may be attained if it is changed to a fast release formulation.

In India where plasma monitoring of drug levels is restricted to only a very few centres, the clinician has no other option but to depend upon the informations provided by drug firms. However, information on bioavailability of a particular product, in comparison to a standard clinically effective drug formulation, is rarely available. In the absence of this data, the clinician usually has no answer to the query 'will the drug get to its site of action in optimal therapeutic concentrations ?' The problem can only be resolved if the clinician insists or scrutinizing its bioavailability data before prescribing a particular drug product.

3

BIOAVAILABILITY STUDIES IN MAN: PHARMACOKINETIC CONSIDERATIONS

Dr. S. K. Garg*

INTRODUCTION

The inter-individual variation in biologic response in patients following administration of same drug can be due to number of factors. Among these, bioavailability can play an important role, which often goes unrecognized. In fact, the time required for absorption of a drug and the amount of the drug absorbed are the two parameters which directly influence the speed of onset and the intensity of drugs pharmacological effects, hence these two parameters must be quantified using bioavailability studies which determine/rate and extent of drug available in systemic circulation.

Generally, bioavailability of a drug product is determined by comparison with a reference preparation in the solution form or another brand of the drug which is known to be well absorbed when taken orally.

To study the bioavailability of drugs, samples should be taken from a location where drug exert their therapeutic effect, since it is not possible to take sample from the site of action, it is usually the general circulation (*i.e.* venous or arterial blood) or the urine. For some drugs, the bioavailability study should be carried out at other levels, *i.e.* in case with locally acting preparations and with substances which act in the gastrointestinal lumen.

In bioavailability studies the pharmacokinetic data obtained should make certain acceptable standards, which would guarantee, as much as possible, that equivalent drugs and different batches of the same drugs would have similar characteristics concerning their therapeutic effects[1].

Usually, bioavailability studies are carried out on healthy subjects and not often in patients due to lack of knowledge of the influence of illness on bioavailability. These investigation should also be carried out in parallel with in vitro tests for the speed of disintegration/degradation and also speed of dissolution to show that correlation exist between in vitro tests and studies performed in man[2].

In healthy human volunteers or in patients the bioavailability studies should be carried out as defined by Helsinki declaration[3]. The procedure

Professor, Department of Pharmacology, Postgraduate Institute of Medical Education and Research, Chandigarh-160 012 (INDIA).

followed for each study should be approved by an expert committee/ethics committee which would have a task to verify that the procedure conforms with the allowed moral standards for experiments to be carried out on human subjects. Both the healthy volunteers and patients who have agreed to participate in these study should be fully informed of the objectives pursued by the study and the conditions under which the study will be carried out, they should give their informed consent in writing and unreservedly, they should be made aware that all necessary protection measures will be taken to ensure their well being[4].

Following methods can be employed to access whether pharmaceutically equivalent products are therapeutically equivalent to one another in order to be considered interchangeable.

1. Comparative bioavailability studies in humans.
2. Comparative pharmacodynamic studies in humans.
3. Comparative clinical trials.
4. In vitro studies for disintegration and dissolution tests.

Bioavailability studies are designed to compare the in vivo performances of a test pharmaceutical product with that of a standard/reference pharmaceutical product. Following aspects should be taken into care for carrying out bioavailability study in man.

1. Investigational product.
2. Selection of subjects/volunteers.
3. Study design.
4. Sample size.
5. Choice of reference standard.
6. Choice of pharmacokinetic parameters.

1. Investigational Products

The test product should meet following requirements:

○ The investigational/test product for bioavailability study should be identical to the reference standard to be used.

○ The content of active drug substance(s) in the test and reference standard should not differ by more than + 5%.

○ The samples of test product should ideally be taken from a industrial scale batches or a small scale production batch provided it is not less than 10% of the size of full scale production batch.

○ Potency and in-vitro dissolution and disintegration characteristic of both test and reference standard must be ascertained prior to starting the bioavailability study.

○ If the test active metabolite is also pharmacologically active then both active drug and active metabolite should be studied.

○ If the active drug substance in the investigational product and reference standard is not possible to measure than the major biotransformation product/metabolite should be measured.

2. Selection of Subjects/Volunteer

The population for bio-availability studies should be homogeneous as far as possible to avoid variability other than in the pharmaceutical product. Therefore, generally these studies are performed in healthy volunteers.

For inclusion and exclusion criteria should be taken into consideration in selecting healthy volunteers for study.

Criteria for inclusion

○ Subjects of either sex.
○ Age between 20 to 50 years.
○ Body weight within normal range as per accepted life tables.
○ Non smokers.
○ No history of alcohol or drug abuse.
○ Volunteers should be screened for suitability by medical history, physical examination, haematological and biochemical tests and values should be within normal limits.

Criteria for exclusion

○ Children
○ Pregnant women
○ Women breast feeding
○ Individuals known to have certain enzyme deficiencies
○ Non-cooperative and inconsistent individuals
○ Individuals in which study drug has not been shown to be harmless and efficacious

Generally bioavailability study should be carried out in healthy volunteers. In case, the test product is known to cause adverse effects which may be considered unacceptable for inclusion of healthy volunteers. The bioavailability study should be performed on patients, who need the investigational test drug for treatment.

3. Study Design

A cross over design with randomized allocation of subjects is the first choice for bioavailability studies. A washout period between the administration of test drug and reference standard of more than five elimination half lives of the drug is minimum and is extended if the drug is converted to active metabolites with longer elimination half life.

Following are the general requirements in relation to protocol design for bioavailability study:

○ Test conditions should be such to have minimum intra and inter subject variability.

○ Avoid bias in results.

○ Restrictions of intake of alcohol, caffeine and citrus juices.

○ Test drug and reference standard ingested same time of the day with same volume of fluid.

○ Test drug and reference standard usually administered in fasting state, (*i.e.* overnight fast) but drug which causes irritation on empty stomach is given with standardized food. Drugs which are expected to increase the bioavailability of drug with food or entirely new moeity should be studied in both fasting and fed conditions.

○ Blood samples should be collected for minimum period of five elimination half-lives of the drug at different time intervals with 3-4 samples in the absorption phase and 4-5 samples during elimination phase for drugs which follow one compartment model while for drugs which follow two compartment model also 2-3 samples during distribution phase.

Special Considerations

(*i*) For drugs which cause unacceptable adverse events in the volunteers, the drugs which are to be given in very high dose and drugs which are very potent, should be studied in patient only.

(*ii*) For drugs with long half life, a parallel design may be preferable and use of truncated area under curve or a multidose study may be required.

(*iii*) Generally for conventional/fast release formulations or fine tuned controlled/modified release formulations, single dose bioavailability studies are sufficient.

(*iv*) Multidose studies for assessing bioavailability/bioequavalence are required for.

○ Drugs with non linear kinetics.

○ Drugs for which assay sensitivity is too low.

○ Drug combination, if ratio of plasma concentration of individual drug substances is important.

4. Sample Size

The number of subjects required for bioavailability study should be 18-24 but not less than 12 subjects in a crossover study.

5. Choice of Reference Standard

Following reference standard should be selected for comparing bioequivalence of the investigational/test drug.

Category or Test Drug	Reference Standard
○ New drug of new drug in any pharmaceutical product.	Solution or suspension of the new drug.
○ New formulation of marketed product.	Approved pharmaceutical product in the market.
○ Controlled/modified release formulation	Approved controlled release product of multinational company or approved conventional formulation
○ Combination drug product	Single ingredient drug product or combination drug product of multinational company.

6. Choice of Pharmacokinetic Parameters

Following pharmacokinetic parameters should be assessed for comparing the bioavailability of a drug.

Conventional Formulations

Peak plasma concentration (C_{max}), Time to reach peak plasma concentration (T_{max}) and Area under the time plasma concentration curve (AUC) should be calculated. The C_{max} and T_{max} characterize the rate of absorption, while AUC serves as the characteristic for the extent of absorption.

Controlled Release Formulation

The area under the time plasma concentration curve (AUC), mean Reseidence Time (MRT) and Mean Absorption Time (MAT) should be calculated. The AUC serves as a characteristic of the extent of absorption while MRT and MAT are the appropriate rate characteristics.

Multiple Dose Study

The Plateau Time (PT), Half Value Duration (HVD), Time above the average concentration (Tabove Cav), Percent Peak-Trough Fluctuation (% PTF), Percentage Swing (%S) and the percentage AUC Fluctuations (% AUCF) are the recommended parameters to characterize the rate and extent of absorption of a drug.

Calculating of Pharmacokinetic Parameters

Different pharmacokinetic parameters used for assessing bioavailability of a drug can be calculated from the plasma/serum concentration-time curve of the drug as follows:

Peak Blood/Plasma Concentration (C_{max})

The mean value of the actual blood/plasma peak concentration of the drug in each volunteer/patient gives C_{max}.

Time to Reach Peak Blood/Plasma Concentration (T_{max})

The mean value of the time at which the peak blood/plasma concentration of the drug is achieved in each volunteer/patient gives T_{max}.

Area Under Blood/Plasma Time Concentration Curve (AUC)

AUC is the measure of quantity of the drug in the body. Following two methods are used to determine the AUC:

1. **Trapezoidal Rule:** A blood level time curve can be described by a series of trapezoids that are determined by each concentration time point. The area of a trapezoid is equal to one half the product of the sum of the concentrations and the time difference.

   Suppose the concentrations of Drug A in plasma at different time intervals in a volunteer are as follows:

TABLE 1

Sample No.	Time (h)	Plasma Concentration (µg/ml)
1.	0.0	0.0
2.	1.0	4.0
3.	2.0	7.0
4.	3.0	13.0
5.	4.0	18.0
6.	6.0	14.0
7.	9.0	9.0
8.	12.0	6.0
9.	24.0	0.5

For calculating AUC of the data of Table 1 by trapezoid rule will be as follows :

$$AUC_{0-24} = (0 + 4 \times 1 - 0) + (4 + 7 \times 2 - 1) + (7 + 13 \times 3 - 2) +$$
(µg/ml.h) $(13 + 18 \times 4 - 3) + (18 + 14 \times 6 - 4) + (14 + 9 \times 9 - 6)$
$$(9 + 6 \times 12 - 9) + (6 + 0.5 \times 24 - 12)/2$$

$$AUC_{0-24} = 4 + 11 + 20 + 31 + 64 + 69 + 45 + 78/2$$
(µg/ml.h)

$$AUC_{0-24} = 322/2 = 161$$
(µg/ml.h)

The remaining or rest area *i.e.* $AUC_{24-\infty}$ is calculated by dividing the last plasma level point by elimination rate constant (Kel or β) under the assumption that this point is beyond the absorptive and distributive phase on the terminal slope of the plasma level curve. The sum of AUC_{0-24} and $AUC_{24-\infty}$ will give $AUC_{0-\infty}$.

2. **Determination of AUC from Blood/Plasma Level Equations:** If the blood/plasma level-time curve of a particular drug in a certain dose size is available, the AUC can be calculated according to following equations.

For intravascular route of administration

$$AUC_{0-\infty} = \frac{D}{Kel.Vd} \text{ (µg/ml.h)}$$

$$AUC_{0-\infty} = \frac{D}{Cl_{tot}}$$

where D—Dose, Kel—elimination rate constant, Vd—volume of distribution, Cl_{tot}—total clearance).

For extravascular route of administration

$$AUC_{0-\infty} = \frac{D.f}{Kel.Vd}$$

$$AUC_{0-\infty} = \frac{D.f}{Cl_{tot}}$$

where *f* is the fraction of drug absorbed.

From AUC the bioavailability (*f*) of a drug and also relative bioavailability (RBA) can be determined by the following equations.

$$f = \frac{AUC_{0-\infty} \text{ oral (mg / ml.h) . Div. (mg)}}{AUC_{0-\infty} \text{ iv (mg / ml.h).D oral (mg)}}$$

S. K. Garg

$$RBA = \frac{AUC_{0-\infty} \text{ oral TD (mg / ml.h)} . D_{SD} \text{ (mg)}}{AUC_{0-\infty} \text{ SD (mg / ml.h)} . D_{TD} \text{ (mg)}}$$

where D is dose of the drug; TD—test drug; SD—standard drug)

Mean Residence Time (MRT)

MRT is calculated by dividing area under moment curve ($AUMC_{0-\infty}$) by area under curve ($AUC_{0-\infty}$).

$$MRT = \frac{AUMC_{0-\infty}}{AUC_{0-\infty}}$$

$AUMC_{0-t}$ is calculated by determining the AUC_{0-t} from the product of time and concentration against the time and $AUMC_{t-\infty}$ is calculated by dividing the last plasma/blood time concentration product by elimination rate constant (Kel or B) and the sum of these two *i.e.* AUC_{0-t} and $AUMC_{t-\infty}$ will be the $AUMC_{0-\infty}$. From Table 1 data the product of time-concentration at different time intervals will be as given in Table 2.

TABLE 2

Time (h)	Product of Time Concentration
0.0	0.0
1.0	2.0
2.0	11.0
3.0	20.0
4.0	31.0
6.0	64.0
9.0	69.0
12.0	45.0
24.0	78.0

Calculate AUC from the product of time concentration against the time. This will give $AUMC_{0-24}$. Dividing the last product of time concentration *i.e.* 78 at 24h by Kel or β will be $AUMC_{24-\infty}$ and the sum of $AUMC_{0-24}$ and $AUMC_{24-\infty}$ will give $AUMC_{0-\infty}$.

Mean Absorption Time (MAT)

This is calculated by the following formula.

$$MAT = MRT \text{ (oral)} \quad MT \text{ (iv)}$$

Plateau Time (PT)

This refers to time span of one dosing interval or dosing cycle *e.g.* 24 hours, during which the serum/plasma drug concentration deviate from the maximum concentration by less than a clinically specified differences or percentage. In case of controlled release theophylline formulation, the PT refers to the during which the concentration exceeds 75% of the maximum concentration and also denoted by T75% C_{max} (See Fig. 1).

Half Value Duration (HVD)

This refers to time span of one dosing interval or dosing cycle 24 hours, during which the serum/plasma drug concentration deviate by 50% from the maximum concentration (Fig. 1). HVD for some drugs may correspond to the plateau time.

Time Above the Average Concentration (Tabove C_{av})

This refers to time span of one dosing interval or dosing cycle 24 hours during which the serum/plasma drug concentration remainis above the average concentration (C_{av}) of one dosing interval or dosing cycle (Fig. 1). The average concentration (C_{av}) is calculated by dividing the AUC of one dosing interval or dosing cycle by dose time interval.

Percentage Peak-Trough Fluctuation (% PTF)

Peak-trough fluctuation relates the peak-tough concentration difference of the drug during one dosing interval to the average concentration (C_{av}).

$$\%PTF = \frac{100(C_{max} - C_{min})}{C_{av}}$$

Percentage Swing (% S)

Swing relates the peak-trough concentration difference of the drug during one dosing interval to the minimum or trough concentration.

$$\%S = \frac{100(C_{max} - C_{min})}{C_{mun}}$$

Area Under Curve Fluctuation (AUCF)

AUCF is based on partial AUC's over one dosing interval. Hence, AUCF relates the difference between AUC above average and below average to the AUC during one dosing interval.

$$\%AUCF = \frac{100 \ (above \ C_{av}) - AUC \ (below \ C_{av})}{AUC}$$

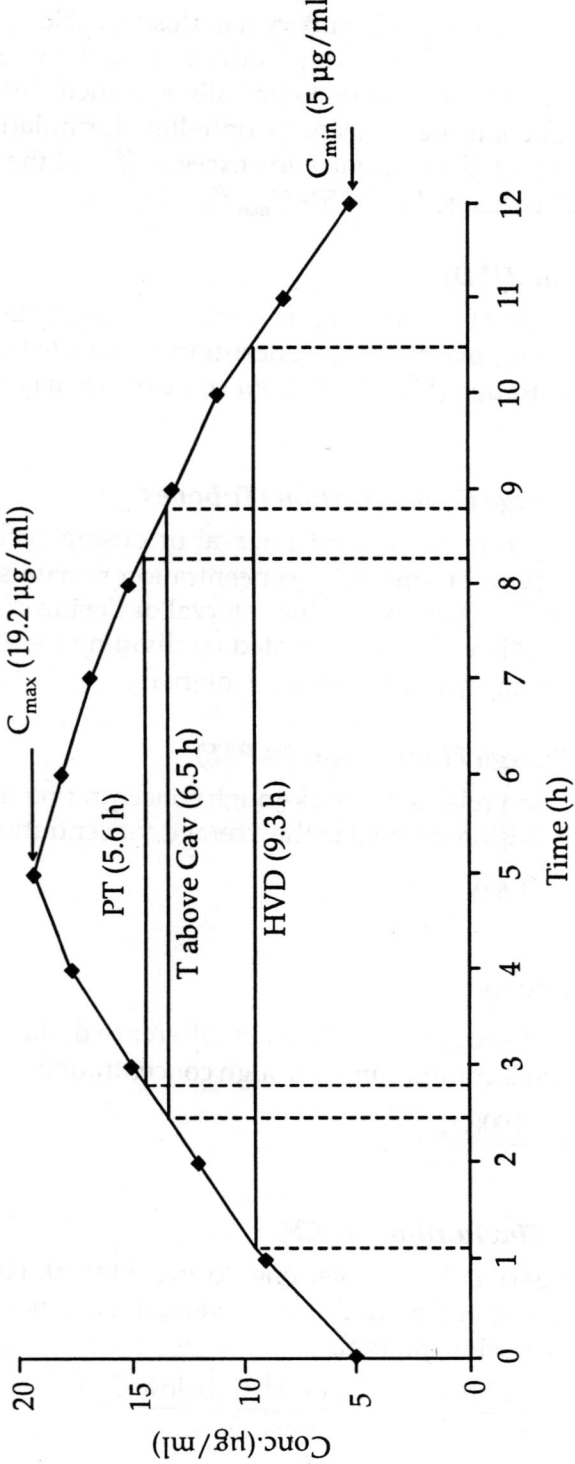

Fig. 1

The plateau time, the time above average concentration and peak trough fluctuation parameters are considered to be rate characteristic of the drug, while Swing and AUCF measures the extent of fluctuation of the plasma/serum concentration of the drug at steady state. With Conventional/Fast releasing formulation at steady state generally there is great extent of fluctuations in swing and AUFC, since these formulation are quickly absorbed when administered orally to give higher peak plasma/serum concentration of the drug followed by rapid elimination of drug by first order kinetics leading to a lower trough concentration, thereby causing much greater fluctuations as compared to sustained/controlled release formulations, where the rate of absorption of drug will be slower and over a long period, thereby leading to lower peak plasma/serum concentration and higher trough concentration causing less fluctuations.

REFERENCES

1. Koch-weser, J. (1974). Bioavailability of drugs. *New Engl. J. Med.*, **291**: 233-237.
2. Ritschel, W. A. (1974). Bioavailability testing and clinical significance. Pharma. *Acta. Helv.*, **49**: 77-83.
3. Azarnoff, D. L. (1972). Physiologic factors in selecting human volunteers for drug studies. *Clin. Pharmacol. Ther.*, **13**: 796-802.
4. Moris, R. C. (1972). Guidelines for accepting volunteers: consent, ethical implications and the function of a pear review. *Clin. Pharmacol. Ther.*, **13**: 782-795.

SELECTED READING MATERIALS

Brodie, B. B. and Heller, W. M. (1972). Bioavailability of drugs. Proceedings of the conference on bioavailability of drugs, S-Karger, Basel-Munich-Paris-London-New York-Sydney.

Cabana, B. E. (1976). Importance of biopharmaceutics and pharamcokinetics in clinical medicine. *Arzneim Forsch*, **26**: 151.

Dittert, L. W. and Disanto, A. R. (1973). Bioavailability of drug products. *J. Am. Med. Assoc.* NS, **13**: 421.

Kaplan, S. A. and Jack, M. L. (1977). Utility of bioavailability studies in drug development. Drug Develop. *Ind. Pharma.*, **3**: 39.

Wagner, J. G. (1976). Pharmacokinetics and bioavailability. *Triangle*, **14**: 101.

Wagner, J. G. (1976). An overview of the analysis and interpretation of bioavailability studies in man. *Arzneim. Forch.*, **26**: 105.

Wolen, R. L. Rubin. A., Rodda, B., Ridolfo, A. and Gruber, C. (1974). Problems associated with bioavailability and dosage regimen studies in man. *J. Pharmacokint. Biopharm.* **2**: 365-377.

4

METHOD OF SAMPLE PREPARATION AND HPLC ANALYSIS OF SOME COMMON DRUGS FROM BIOLOGICAL FLUIDS

Dr. Vivek R. Dhole and Mr. B. Sitharaman*

INTRODUCTION

HPLC system has several facilities which can be utilised to detect the drugs in the biological materials, such as blood, urine etc. Selective detection of drugs relative to the matrix is achieved by selecting the suitable stationary phase or even the composition of the mobile phase can be altered to achieve such separation. The sample preparation involves several factors, including the nature of the sample blood, urine etc. the condition of the sample, and concentration level of the drug. Interference from the matrix components is maximum when the concentration of the drug is very low and special sample preparation is often required. Conditions of the sample also affects such assay, *e.g.* recoveries from fresh blood and the haemolysed one may not be similar by the same sample preparation method.

FILTRATION METHODS

The most common method for clearing the sample is by filtration, either by the filter paper or sintered glass crucible. The filter itself is first washed with the solvent. The solvents are selected in such a way so as to dissolve the maximum possible amount of the solute of interest. However, if solutes of interest are present at a very low concentrations, *i.e.*, in ppm levels, then a significant amount of them may be lost because of their adsorption on the matrix solid material that is being removed from the sample by way of filtration. Such problems of adsorption are considerably reduced if the contaminating solid material is removed by centrifugation.

PRECIPITATION AND CENTRIFUGATION TECHNIQUES

Drug which is physically or chemically bound, to the surface of the proteins must be released, then the protein is precipitated to leave the drug in aqueous solution. The protein may be degraded by strong acids or enzymes or

Toshniwal Instruments (I) Pvt. Ltd. D-96, MIDC, 'C' Road, Satpur, Nasik-422 007.

precipitated by some chemicals like ammonium sulphate or removed by ultra filtration. But some drugs are susceptible to protein degradation methods and sometimes precipitation and ultrafilteration can lead to losses because of their binding to the proteins. A single procedure cannot work for recovery of all types of drugs from different types of substrate materials. Direct injections of deproteinised solutions are made and analysed on HPLC system by using the polar mobile phase. The biological fluid is mixed and shaken with methanol or acetonitrile and centrifuged to remove the precipitated proteins and the supernatant liquid is used for injection. The proteins are separated out before injection to protect the sample valve and analytical column from irreversible contamination and clogging. Urine can be similarly treated to remove the salts. The centrifugation method thus requires a special micro centrifuge apparatus, it has several merits over the other purification methods. Firstly, there is no filter device on which trace components of the sample can be lost due to adsorption, secondly the sample volume is not changed during the solid removal. Small glass centrifuge tubes are used but if strongly polar trace materials/solutes are present, they may be adsorbed by the polar hydroxyl groups on the wall of the glass tubes, in such cases the tube wall can be deactivated by reacting the surface hydroxyl groups with appropriate alkyl silane groups. In the centrifugation method, nature of the matrix, nature of the solutes, degree of adsorption of the solute with the matrix, choice of suitable solvent for the maximum solubility of the solute in the solvent play the major role in achieving the maximum percent recovery of the solute from the matrix.

EXTRACTION AND CONCENTRATION TECHNIQUE

Because of the limited detector sensitivity, there is very often a need of extracting and then concentrating the analyte solution while determining the traces specially in the Biomedical, Foresic and environmental samples. Solvent extraction is the most popular approach, as several parameters can be modified to optimise the extent of extraction. Such modifications include changing the polarity of the organic solvent, the pH and ionic nature and strength of the aqueous phase and use of ion pairing agents. After extracting the sample by suitable solvent the organic extract may be directly injected into the column after using the centrifugation or filtration methods or the analyte solution is further concentrated by evaporation, where the solutes are relatively sufficiently non volatile compared to the solvents in which they are dissolved. For the oxidisable compounds the evaporation can be carried out in presence of nitrogen and for thermally labile compounds also have to be concentrated by evaporation below the thermal decomposition temperature.

LYOPHILISATION

It is a similar technique but it is evaporation at reduced temperature under vacuum. Some aqueous samples can be frozen and the vapour pressure of the ice is sufficient to produce a relatively faster rate of evaporation. Also, where, the analytes have sufficiently high vapour pressures at room temperatures, to cause loss of solute by normal evaporation procedures, the Lyophilisation method is used. This method is gentler than the evaporation and hence is being used for the samples of biological origin and the thermally labile analytes and for substances like protesin which denature easily. Special equipment are available for Lyophilisation.

UTILITY OF GUARD COLUMNS

A short guard column is generally introduced between the injector and the analytical column. It is packed with the same material as the analytical column with a larger particle size to minimize the pressure drop and is replaced after some specific duration due to contamination. The ratio of guard column volume to analytical column volume should be around 1 : 20, which keeps band broadening to the minimum, while maintaining sufficient capacity to retain the impurities. Usually the guard column is introduced to increase the life of the analytical column by removing the particulate matter and impurities from the solvent components that bind irreversibly to the stationary phase. Also, in liquid chromatography the guard column serves to saturate the mobile phase with the stationary phase so that the losses of the solvent from the analytical column are minimised. Thus the guard column protects the more expensive analytical column. But such a device introduces an extra column volume in the chromatographic system, causing peak dispersion and thus impair resolution where just a marginal level of resolution is achieved with the selected phase system.

SOLID PHASE EXTRACTION (SPE) PROCEDURE

The Solid Phase Extraction (SPE) method involves the use of the short inert plastic cartridge (tube) packed with an adosorbent, usually a reversed phase or an ion exchange resin. The particle size is usually larger than that used in the LC analytical column to avoid the pressure drop and to ensure the reasonable permeability. Depending upon the type of application, a wide variety of materials can be chosen as the adsorbent, which may range from silica gel, reverse phase material, ion exchange resins or affinity packings. Thus, solid phase extraction is essentially an extraction process which comprises a solid and a liquid phase. The components of interest and the matrix interference are in the liquid phase. SPE is based on the principle that the components of interest, mainly organic compounds, are mainly retained on the solid adsorbent placed in a disposable cartridge. The interfering components and solvent molecules (matrix) are not retained and are washed with the suitable solvent. The remaining interfering components are removed from the adsorbent by elution with other suitable solvent. Finally the analyte is removed from the absorbent by elution with the suitable solvent, or mobile phase.

The main objectives of SPE are removal of interfering matrix components and selective separation and concentration of analytes. Enrichment can increase the detection sensitivity of the analytes by the factor of 100 to 5000. Such an enrichment is useful for trace level qualitative and quantitative analysis of analytes and also the separation from interfering matrix components.

SPE involves four steps:

(a) Conditioning of the sorbent: Usually effected by passing the solvent prior to sample injection, so that the sorbent in the SPE cartridge can interact with the sample. This process is also called as salvation.

(b) Sample injection: After conditioning the adsorbent bed should not run dry, otherwise salvation is non effective. Then, the sample solution is forced through the sorbent of the cartridge at about 3 ml/min flow rate. The components of interest (analytes) are adsorbed by the sorbent.

(c) Washing of the absorbent: It is being achieved by using some solvents to remove undesired matrix components from the cartridge.

(d) Elution: Elution is effected by selectively desorbing the compounds of interest from the sorbent and collecting the cartridge effluent.

SPE has become a safe, powerful and fast means of sample preparation having applications in the environmental, pharmaceutical, food, forensic and biochemical analyses, *e.g.*, isolation of analytes such as PCBs, Pesticides, PAHs, Drugs, Vitamins and dyes from matrices such as water, soil, tablets, blood, urine, food stuffs, vegetables and fruits is effected.

Automatic Solid Phases Extraction System

A typical of such system comprises of auto sampler, SPE pump, SPE cartridge, switching valves, separate pumps for binary high pressure gradient HPLC system, an analytical HPLC column and suitable detector (usually UV detector) A typical of such system is manufactured as UNEXAS system by M/s. Knauer, Germany, which is being marketed in India by M/s. Chemito Instruments Pvt. Ltd., Mumbai. Some popular and typical examples of SPE reported in the literature are as follows:

(1) Tetra hydro cannabinol carboxylic acid from urine.
(2) Tricyclic antidepressant drugs from blood serum.

(3) Amphetamine codeine and morphine from blood.

(4) Individual components in different groups e.g. aromatic amines, phenols, PCBs. PAHs and pesticides from water and soil (environmental) samples.

(5) Catecholamines in urine sample.

(6) Analysis of caffeine in cola samples.

(7) Benzalkonium chloride from waste water.

(8) Mycotoxins from apple juice.

There are several such applications reported on SPE-HPLC analysis.

HPLC Systems for Commonly Used Drugs

HPLC is a very popular technique for the analysis of various classes of drugs in pharma industries. They can be analysed as such or after extraction from blood, plasma or tissue samples, after using some of the clean up as described above. The detection of these drugs are usually done by a UV detector or by using diode array or fluorescence detector. Some common examples are given below.

HPLC Analytical Data

Drug	Column	Mobile Phase	Detection
Amphetamines and other stimulants	C-18	0.2 m of phosphoric acid and 0.1 m of diethyl amine in 10% MeOH	UV at 250 nm
Antihistamines	Silica	Methanolic amn. Perchlorate (10 mM, pH = 6.7)	UV at 254 nm
Barbiturates	C-18	Methanol : 0.1 M sod. dihydro-gen phosphate (40 : 60)	UV at 216 nm
Benzodiazepines	C-18	Methanol : Water : phosphate buffer (55 : 25 : 20)	UV at 240 nm
Penicillins Sodium Ampicillin Sodium Oxacillin Sodium Cloxacillin Sodium Flucloxacillin	C-18	Methanol/Water 1% $NaHCO_3$ 45 : 55 : 0.8	UV at 220 nm
Analgesics Propoxyphene Acetaminophen Codeine	C-18	Acetonitrile/0.05 M KH_2PO_4 Containing 0.02% Triethylamine 40 : 60 : pH 3.0	UV at 254 nm
Antibiotics Chloramphenicol and its Metabolite	C-8	Acetonitrile/Methanol 20 mM H_3PO_4 Containing 0.02% Triethylamine 6 : 20 : 74	UV at 254 nm

Antibacterials Trimethoprim Sulfamethoxazole Ciprofloxacin	C-18	0.1% Triethylamine in 20% Acetonitrile pH-9. Phosphate Buffer/Acetonitrile/ Methanol 81 : 5 : 14	UV at 254 nm Fluorescence EX. 270 nm EM. 440 nm
Hydrocortisone	C-18	Sodium Acetate Buffer/ (0.05 ml/litre pH 8) Acetonitrile 77 : 23	UV at 254 nm
Ibuprofen	C-18	Acetonitrile/Water/Glacial Acetic Acid 45 : 55 : 0.32	UV at 240 nm
Theophylline Caffeine Chloramphenicol Phenytoin	C-8	Acetonitrile/Water 20 : 80	UV at 208 nm

There are several such HPLC methods reported for the analysis of drugs in pharma and biomedical applications and day by day field of HPLC analytical technique is growing enormously.

5

APPLICATION OF HPLC FOR THE ANALYSIS OF BIOLOGICAL SAMPLES AND DRUGS

Anil K Ghosh*, Nilima Biswas* and Subhobrata Sengupta*

INTRODUCTION

High performance chromatography (HPLC) has been in use since late 1960s and now a days this instrument is considered to be an essential tool for any analytical laboratory[1]. HPLC is of itself not a new method, but rather a refinement of known methods combined with greater instrumental complexity and precession. Consequently, pump systems providing constant flow rates of mobile phase at high pressure, pressure-stable column filling materials replacing conventional soft gels, used in ordinary liquid chromatography and evenly packed columns with increased reproducibility were developed. The successful application of HPLC as a quantitative analytical method requires great care in the choice and purity of the solvent, a highly constant flow rate, and continual checks of column performance. A typical HPLC apparatus (Fig. 1) consists of a high pressure pumping system (which drives the **mobile phase**), a sample applicator (injector), a column (**stationary phase**), and a detector. It is also possible to include a fraction collector and/or a personal computer for data processing. Automatic injector is desirable if the instrument is to be employed for routine analytical or preparative purposes.

If we look at a HPLC system, we find the instrument is composed of several modules each with its own function (Fig. 1). A sample, to be analysed, is normally introduced into the system via an *injector* from which it is forced by a flowing stream of solvent, commonly known as *mobile phase*, through a narrow (0.009 inch i.d.) bore transport tube to the *column*. The column is a large (2-8 mm i.d.) tube containing very small but tightly packed silica particles (2-50 µm), known as stationary phase. The sample, consisting of different components, separates as a result of differential adhering or diffusion for stationary phase. Thus, as the mobile phase is forced through the chromatographic bed, a sample is separated into various zones of sample components, commonly known as *bands*. The bands continue to might through the bed, eventually pass out of the column, known as *elution* and

*Indian Institute of Chemical Biology, 4, Raja S.C. Mullick Road, Calcutta-700 032.

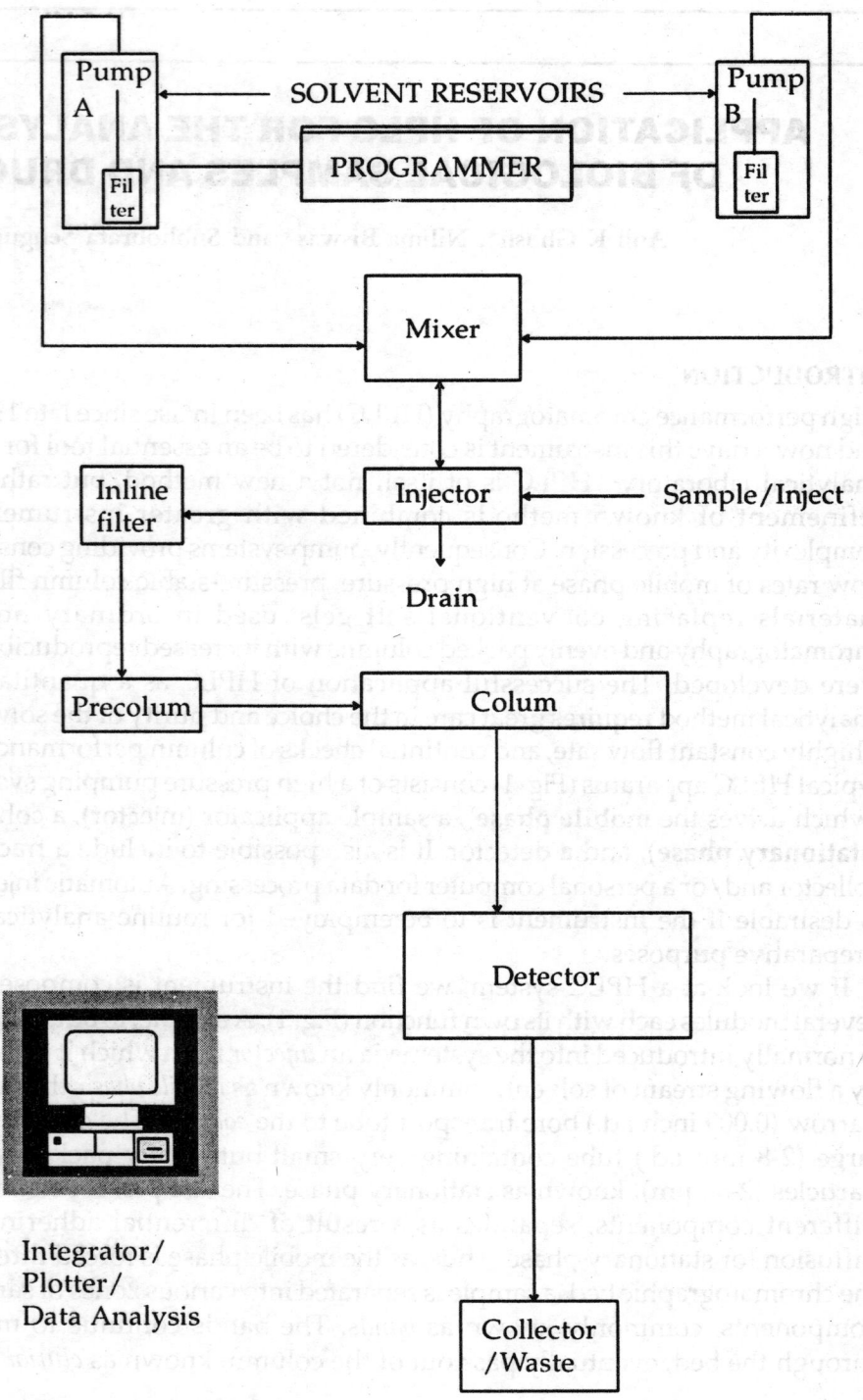

Fig. 1: Basic Design of a Typical HPLC System

pass through any one or more detectors. The detector then provides signal to the recording device. The recorder tracing from the elution of a single band is known as a peak and the collection of peaks resulting from an injected sample comprise the *chromatogram*. Peaks are normally identified by their *retention time*, which is the time required to elute the corresponding band from the column. The peaks on the recorder resembles a Gaussian (bell-shaped) curve. So a band in the column features a zone of material that is concentrated in the centre and more dilute at the edges. The theoretical *plate number (N)* is a characteristic property of every column which describes the deviation of a band around the centre and so it is commonly taken as a measure of column performance. It should be mentioned here that N will not necessarily be the same for systems where the solvent, instrument flow rate, etc. are changed quite often. N measures band spreading in the entire LC system, from injection to detection, and is usually meaningful only when compared to a standard. Plate numbers for well-packed HPLC columns are directly proportional to the column length and inversely proportional to the particle diameter. Since HPLC column materials are made of relatively small tightly packed particles they exhibit high performance in comparison to the conventional chromatographic materials.

ANALYSIS OF BIOLOGICAL SAMPLES

Living cells are highly organised compartments in which varieties of self-regulating chemical reactions are going on. Needless to mention, understanding these chemical reactions is an extremely important task to unravel several biological events, *e.g.* how cells reproduce, grow, maintain viability and eventually why cells die. Among several techniques available now-a-days, for the anlaysis of biological samples HPLC analysis is considered to be most useful since almost all analysis can be handled by a single machine and requires very little sample. Among several applications related to analysis of bio-molecules, HPLC analysis of both small compounds, *e.g.* amino acids, cAMP, S-adenosyl L-methionine (AdoMet) etc. and large polymeric compounds like proteins, peptides, etc., are discussed here.

ESTIMATION OF SMALL BIO-CHEMICALS

Cyclic adenosine 3', 5'-monophosphate (cAMP) is an extremely important bio-molecule which serves as a regulator for varieties of biochemical reactios of animals, micro-organisms and possibly also of higher plants. Trehalose (α-D-glucopyranosyl α-D-Glucopyranoside), an important storage disaccharide is present in a great diversity or organisms ranging form bacteria to plants and mammals[2]. Differential trehalose metabolism including trehalose hydrolysis by trehalase (α, α-trehalose 1-D-glucohydrolase, EC 3.2.1.28) has been shown to be related to morphological differentiation in yeast[3]. Among the two different trehalases, activation of neutral trehalase (NT) is mediated through cAMP dependent protein phosphorylation while the regulation of acid trehalase (AT) activity has been shown to be related to intracellular metabolism of the biological methyl group donor, S-adenosyl-L-methionine (AdoMet)[4]. Consequently development of methodology for monitoring change in intracellular cAMP and AdoMet level throughout the entire yeast life cycle was very much needed. In this regard, a method was developed for the analysis of these two important biochemicals using HPLC[4]. Yeast strain including culture condition and preparation of cell free extract using 0.5 (N) perchloric acid has been described earlier[4].

ANALYSIS OF CAMP AND RELATED COMPOUNDS

HPLC system consisted of two 501 pumps driven by a 680 programmer, 484 LC spectrophotometer and 745B data module (Waters, USA). Analysis was made by an anion-exchange column, Partisil 10 SAX (4.6 × 250 mm, Whatman, England). Mobile phases used were A : 7 mM KH_2PO_4, 7mM KCl, pH 4.0 and B : 250 mM KH_2PO_4, 750 mM KCl, pH 5.0. A binary gradient elution profile was used at a flow rate of 2 ml/min as : 0-5 min, 100% A; 5-25 min, 100% B; 25-35 min, 100% B; and subsequently equilibration of the column was made by passing mobile phase for 35-37 min, 100% A; 37-52 min, 100% A. Samples were detected at an absorbency 254 nm and peaks were analysed, both qualitatively and quantitatively, with respect to standard samples. Peak areas were arbitrary numbers obtained from the 745 B data module print out which was preadjusted to: attenuation = 256, chart speed = 0.25 cm./min. Identification of cAMP peaks were made from the relative comparison of cyclic nucleotide phosphodiesterase treated and untreated samples. For phosphodiesterase treatment, samples (2 ml) were taken in 0.1 M tris-HCl buffer (pH 7.0) containing $MgCl_2$ 10 mM, 2-mercaptoethanol 100 µM and phosphodiesterase 0.1 U and were incubated at 30°C for 30 min. Reaction was stopped by the addition of 0.2 ml of 1.0 N ice-cold perchloric acid. And placed immediately on a ice-bath and kept as such for 1 hour. Thus treated samples exhibited no cAMP peak Sample volume, 10-50 µl, containing 10-100 n mole of cAMP or related compounds, could be detected efficiently using this procedure. Elution time (E_t, min) recorded were as follows : cAMP 4.10, cGMP 6.71, 3' AMP 6.73, ADP 18.11, ATP 33.5, respectively.

ANALYSIS OF ADOMET AND RELATED COMPOUNDS

HPLC system and related techniques were same as described above. HPLC column, Partisil 10SCX (4.6 × 250 mm, Whatman, England), was used. Samples eluted at a flow rate of 0.5 ml/min were detected at 259 nm and other conditions were same as stated above. Mobile phase A was 0.7 ml concentrated NH_4OH per litre of 20% acetonitrile in water and adjusted to pH 3.0 with 88% formic acid and B was 50 mM $(NH_4)_2SO_4$ in mobile phase

A, adjusted to pH 3.0 with concentrated sulphuric acid. Isocratic elution of samples were made using 70% B and 30% A instead of gradient elution as used earlier. Elution time (min) recorded were as follows: AdoMet 15.6, S-adenosyl L-homocysteine 9.06, adenosine 8./6 and adenine 9.9.

AMINO ACID ANALYSIS

Determination of amino acid composition of protein/peptide can be determined using a PICO. TAG work station as per operation manual provided by the manufacturer (Waters, USA). Protein or peptide was hydrolysed and then derivatized by phenyl isothyocyanate (PITC) and was analysed, both qualitatively and quantitatively, using an amino acid analysis column, as reported earlier[5].

Determination of free amino acids of whole blood is very important form the clinical point of view. Hydrolysis of protein/peptide by HCl is not needed here to determine free amino acid composition and so hydrolysis step should be omitted. Same PITC-amino acid analysis protocol, as discussed above, may be used. Low molecular weight compounds including free amino acids were extracted by 0.5 (N) perchloric acid, as stated above. Neutralised amino acid containing solution was then taken directly into the PITC-derivatizing tubes and PITC-amino acids prepared were analyseded, both qualitatively and quantitatively, as discussed above.

Introduction of equivalent among of tributylamine in lieu of triethylamine, appeared to be better for resolving anionic animo acids, *e.g.*, asparticacid, glutamic acid, phosporylated amino acids, etc. (unpublished observatioin). Besides all those, as discussed above, analysis of fermented broth[6], batch standardisation of food products[7], etc. can be made using HPLC.

HPLC OF PROTEIN

Application of HPLC for analysis or purification of protein or peptide samples has undergone a dramatic development in recent years[8, 9]. With the development of recombinant DNA technology, requirement for efficient methodology either for analysis or for purification of the recombinant products became an absolute requirement by the scientists world wide. The progress of gene technology has resulted in a renaissance of protein chemistry. The new analytical and preparative problems that have emerged because of progress of gene technology are mostly solved by HPLC methods. Some of the applications of HPLC in the chemistry of amino acids, peptides and proteins are:

Analytical

O Amino acids analysis,

O Purity control of synthetic peptides and thereby optimisation, of reaction conditions,

○ Identification of multiple forms of proteins,
○ Molecular weight approximation,
○ Peptide mapping,
○ Amino acid sequence analysis of proteins or peptides,
○ Product characterisation after chemical or biochemical modification of enzyme,
○ Determination of enzyme specificity,
○ Metabolism studies.

Preparative

○ Isolation and purification,
○ Purification after chemical synthesis or gene technology,
○ Purification of modified peptides or proteins (*e.g.*, radio actively labelled),
○ Separation of diastereomers.

Various separation modes, normally used for the HPLC of proteins or peptides may be summarised as follows:

(a) Ion-Exchange (IE) HPLC

Proteins or peptides are amphoteric and so can exist in either cationic or anionic form depending upon the pH of the solution. A characteristic parameter of any protein or peptide is their *isoelectricpoint* (pH) at which the net charge is zero. Elution of protein or peptide can be brought about by a *gradient* of increasing ionic strength, a pH gradient, or a combination of both. Columns are mostly made of silica derivatives or hydrophilic organic polymers, such as TSK-PW series columns, the latter being more popular since those can be used at wide range of pH. The best choice for most protein separation problems is a pore size of 300 Å, while for molecules with molecular weight larger than 150,000 a pore size of 1000 Å or more is preferred. Among the anion exchangers, diethylaminoethyl (DEAE), Mono-Q, etc. and among the cation exchangers, sulfopropyl (SP), Mono-S, etc. are available commercially. Scaling up, *e.g.*, selection of stationary phase, pH, etc. may be made using ordinary chromatographic materials before a costly HPLC column is used. Retention mechanism exhibited by the stationary phase here is electrostatic inteactions between functional groups in the molecules and on the surface of the ion exchangers. So a small column can retain relatively larger quantity of protein or peptide and as a result of which purification following this procedure favours association of protein molecules.

(b) Hydrophobic Interaction (HI) and Reversed-Phase (RP) HPLC

Amino acids present in proteins or peptides contain both nonpolar hydrophobic and polar hydrophilic moieties. Most of the hydrophobic moieties of a soluble protein is located inside the three dimensional structure and a few hydrophobic points remains on the surface. These surface hydrophobic points of contacts can lead to adsorption on a non polar stationary phase. Retention mechanisms for both HI - and RP-JPLC are same, the former being relatively milder. The hydrophobic interaction is strong in the presence of high concentration of ions, increasing temperature and weakens with decreasing concentration of ion. During HI-HPLC proteins are taken in semi-saturated ammonium sulphate solution and is applied to the column which is subsequently eluted using a reverse gradient. Commercially available HI-HPLC columns are mostly made from (organic polymeric materials, *e.g.*, TSK-phenyl-5PW, TSK-ether -5P, etc. Besides ammonium sulphate; sodium sulphate, sodium or potassium phosphates, etc. are also used.

In contrast to HI-HPLC, significantly more nonpolar, *i.e.*, more heavily alkylated stationary phases are used in RP-HPLC. So proteins or peptides bind to the matrix even in aqueous buffers of low ionic strength. Commercially available RP-columns are mostly made from silica but columns made of organic polymerised substances are also available. Some of the RP-columns are, Lichrosorb RP-18, µ-BondaPak C18, DeltaPak C4 or-CB or C-18, etc. Since the stationary phase here is more hydrophobic, elution of protein/peptide requires introduction of organic solvent in the eluting mobile phase. Consequently, this procedure is not a very good method for the purification or analysis of peptides, amino acids, etc. RP-HPLC is undoubtedly one of the most efficient methods of separation but HI-HPLC is very good for biologically active proteins. Some of the most important applications of both HPLC procedures are : studies related to protein folding, change in protein conformation, etc.[10].

(c) Gel Permeation (GP) HPLC

GP-HPLC is considered to be a special procedure since, unlike to the procedures mentioned above, there is no interaction between the sample and the stationary phase here. This is also known as size exclusion or gel filtration HPLC. Here separation takes place according to the distribution of size of hydrodyanamic volume of the molecules in a given solvent (mobile phase). Mobile phases mostly used here for the separation of protein samples are aqueous buffers. The column packings are porous solid silica get or rigid organic polymer or resin. Stationary phase particles are mostly spherical with specific porosity through which only certain molecules of known molecular size can enter and as a result of which they are retained longer while other molecules of larger size can bot enter the pores and are eluted earlier (*void volume*). Molecules which enter the pores are eluted (*Elution volume*) as per their size, *i.e.*, the larger molecules are eluted earlier while smaller molecules are eluted latter. Main advantage of this procedure is that elution is rapid and the entire sample is eluted within one column volume. Since the molecules do not come into contact with the surface of the stationary phase, there is no opportunity for conformational changes to take place and so the method is extremely soft and retains very well the biological activity of the proteins. On the other hand, it has two main disadvantages. First, it has a low peak capacity and second, silica or organic stationary phases tend to adsorb proteins through ionic or hydrophobic interactions and so mobile phases used here are mostly higher ionic strength buffers. Use of higher ionic strength buffer is not good for the HPLC system and so the entire system should be thoroughly by HPLC grade water before the system is turned off. Though samples applied here can be recovered in totality but almost 3-5 volume dilution of the sample is normally encountered after elution.

Most enzymes exist as oligomers or protomers and many of them can reversibly dissociate or reassociate in response to effector ligand. Among various post translational protein modifications regulating catalytic function of several enzymes, reversible oligomerisation among enzyme molecules has been shown to be responsible for the regulation of their activities. Among various modes used in HPLC, IE-HPLC favours association among protein molecules while GP-HPLC favours dissociation, possibly because of dilution. Consequently, HPLC has been used extensively to prove above theory using several carbohydrates, *e.g.* cellobiase[11], amyloglucosidase[4], acid trehalase [12, 13].

(d) Affinity HPLC

Retention in affinity HPLC is due to biospecific interactions between sample molecules and affinity ligand bonded on a support. Stationary phases are prepared by the user himself by coupling the appropriate ligand to glass, silica gel or organic polymers. Some of the ligands have a variety of applications, *e.g.*, AMP, protein A, lectins, etc. This method is not very much popular since it requires several steps, *e.g.*, preparation of stationary phase, column packing, etc. before one attempts to use this kind of HPLC.

Analysis of Drugs

Analysis of drug is an extremely important aspect of pharmacological as well as biological research. Determination of amount of drug incorporated into the serum is a standard clinical practice for optimising drug dosages. This is not only very much essential either during treatment with important drugs but also during research and development work on new drug development. By definition drug analysis is the quantitative determination of drugs and their metabolites in biological samples and the interpretation of such data using principles of pharmacokinetics and pharmacodynamics. Needless to mention, since drug monitoring is an important task, almost all major hospitals have established clinical chemistry sections devoted to the analysis of therapeutic drug concentrations. Several techniques *e.g.*, high performance liquid chromatography (HPLC), gas chromatography (GC), ultra violet spectroscopy (UV), radioimmunoassay (RIA), enzyme immuno assay (EIA), etc., are routinely used in any analytical laboratory. Both HPLC and GC are very much practised in most of the clinical laboratories, the former being more versatile. Now-a-days various detectors, *e.g.*, UV-VIS LC spectrophotometer (most common), refractive index, electrochemical, fluorometer, etc., are routinely used during drug analysis. The recent advancement regarding HPLC drug assays from biological samples, or even in a quality control, laboratory attached to a pharmaceutical industry is based on the versatility, efficacy, precision, and speed of this techique. Rapid technological advancements made it possible to employ HPLC as a routine method for both qualitative and quantitative drug analysis.

Preparation of samples for HPLC analysis depends mostly on the chemistry of the drug to be analysed and removal of the contaminants from the sample prior to analysis. This might be simply perchloric acid or solvent extraction, pre- or post-column derivatization, etc. Almost all HPLC modes, *e.g.*, IE-HPLC, RP-HPLC, GP-HPLC, as discussed earlier, are used for drug analysis. Moreover, stationary phase made of bare silica particles, often called normal phase (NP), are also used for the analysis of relatively lipophilic drugs. Among all these modes RP-HPLC is mostly practised in any laboratory. During RP-HPLC, the stationary phase is less polar in comparison to that used in NP-HPLC and so non-polar drugs are well separated by RP-HPLC. Moreover, polar drugs can also be analysed by RP-HPLC either in combination with *ion suppression* or by introducing some *ion pairing* agents. Ion suppression is mostly made by using a mobile phase of low pH so that active functional groups (*e.g.*, -COOH, ArOH, etc.) remainings unionised mostly during analysis. Ion pairing agents for pairing with both acidic (tetrabutyl ammonium phosphate, dibutylamine phosphate) and basic (pentane/hexane/heptane sulfonic acid) functional groups of sample molecules are available commercially. Introduction of these agents in the mobile phase is very much useful for the analysis of a complicated sample containing both polar, non polar and neutral ingredients.

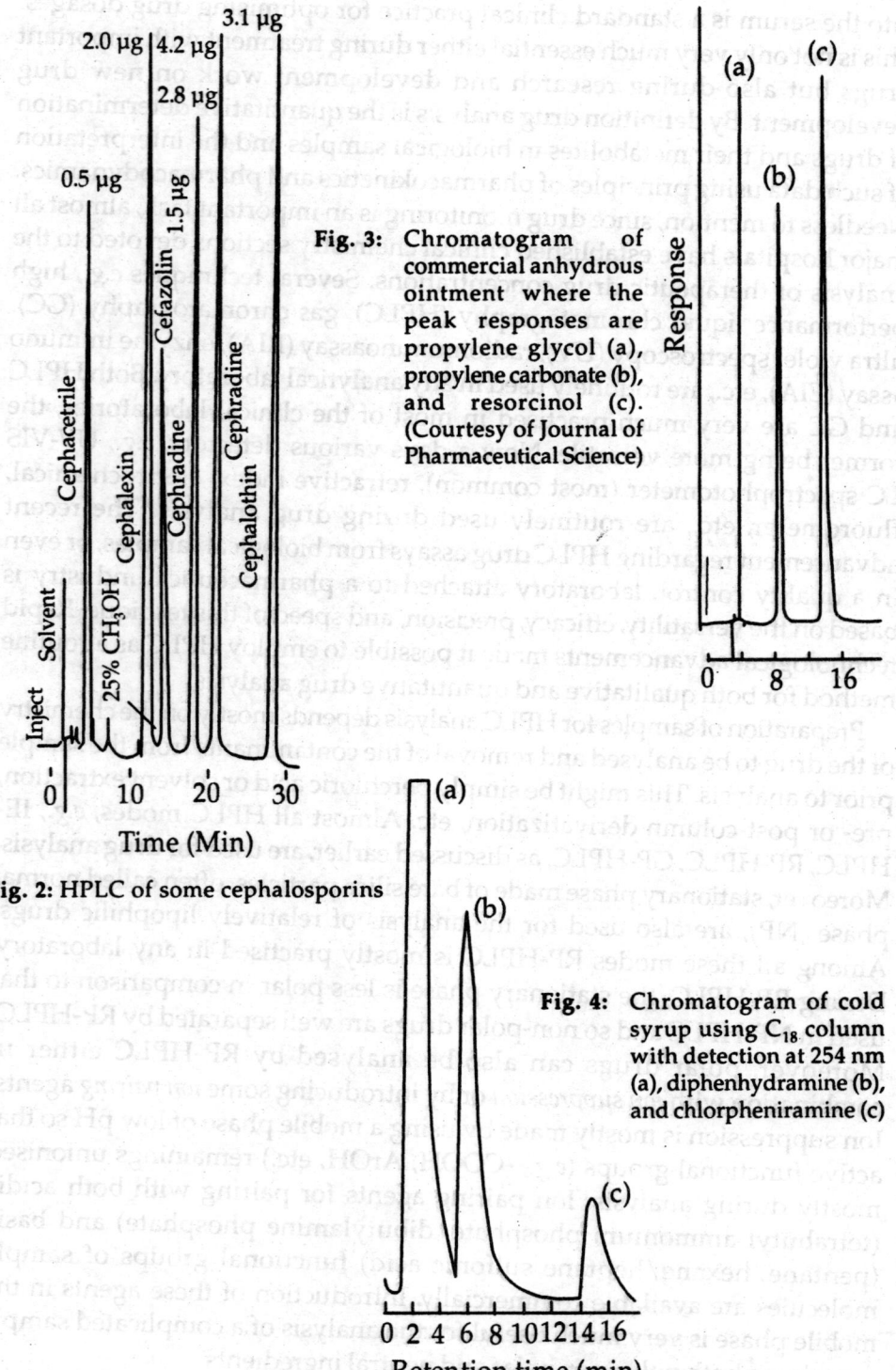

Fig. 3: Chromatogram of commercial anhydrous ointment where the peak responses are propylene glycol (a), propylene carbonate (b), and resorcinol (c). (Courtesy of Journal of Pharmaceutical Science)

Fig. 2: HPLC of some cephalosporins

Fig. 4: Chromatogram of cold syrup using C_{18} column with detection at 254 nm (a), diphenhydramine (b), and chlorpheniramine (c)

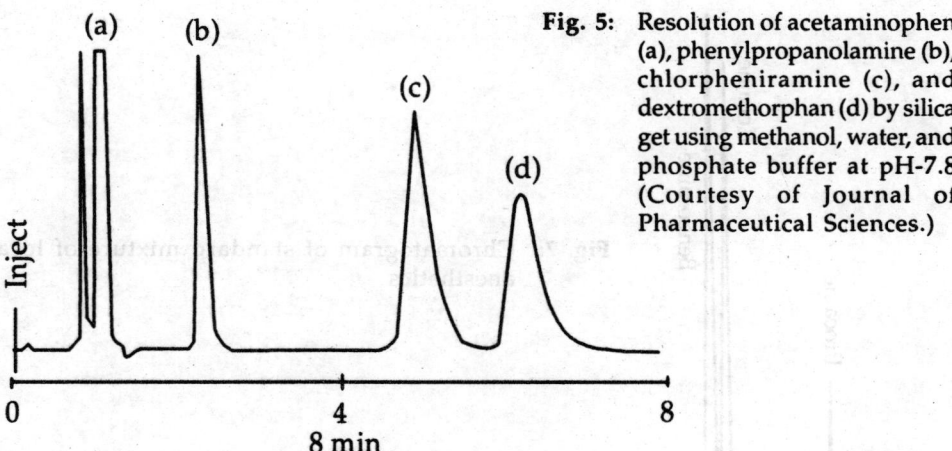

Fig. 5: Resolution of acetaminophen (a), phenylpropanolamine (b), chlorpheniramine (c), and dextromethorphan (d) by silica get using methanol, water, and phosphate buffer at pH-7.8 (Courtesy of Journal of Pharmaceutical Sciences.)

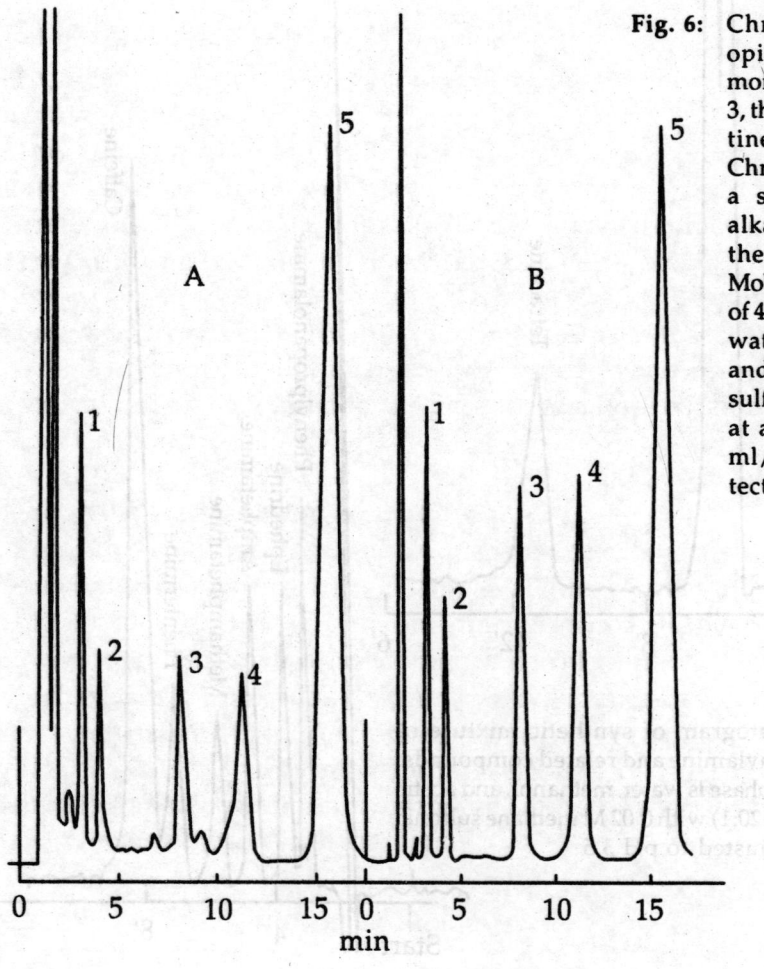

Fig. 6: Chromatogram of opium sample A:1, morphine:2, codeh e; 3, thebaine, 4, naroco-tine;5, papaverine. Chro-matogram of B, a synthetic opium alka-loid mixture of these compounds. Mobile phase consists of 40% methanol, 50% water, 1% acetic acid, and 0.005 M heptane sulfonic acid (pH 3.5) at a flow rate of 2.0 ml/minute. UV de-tection at 254 nm

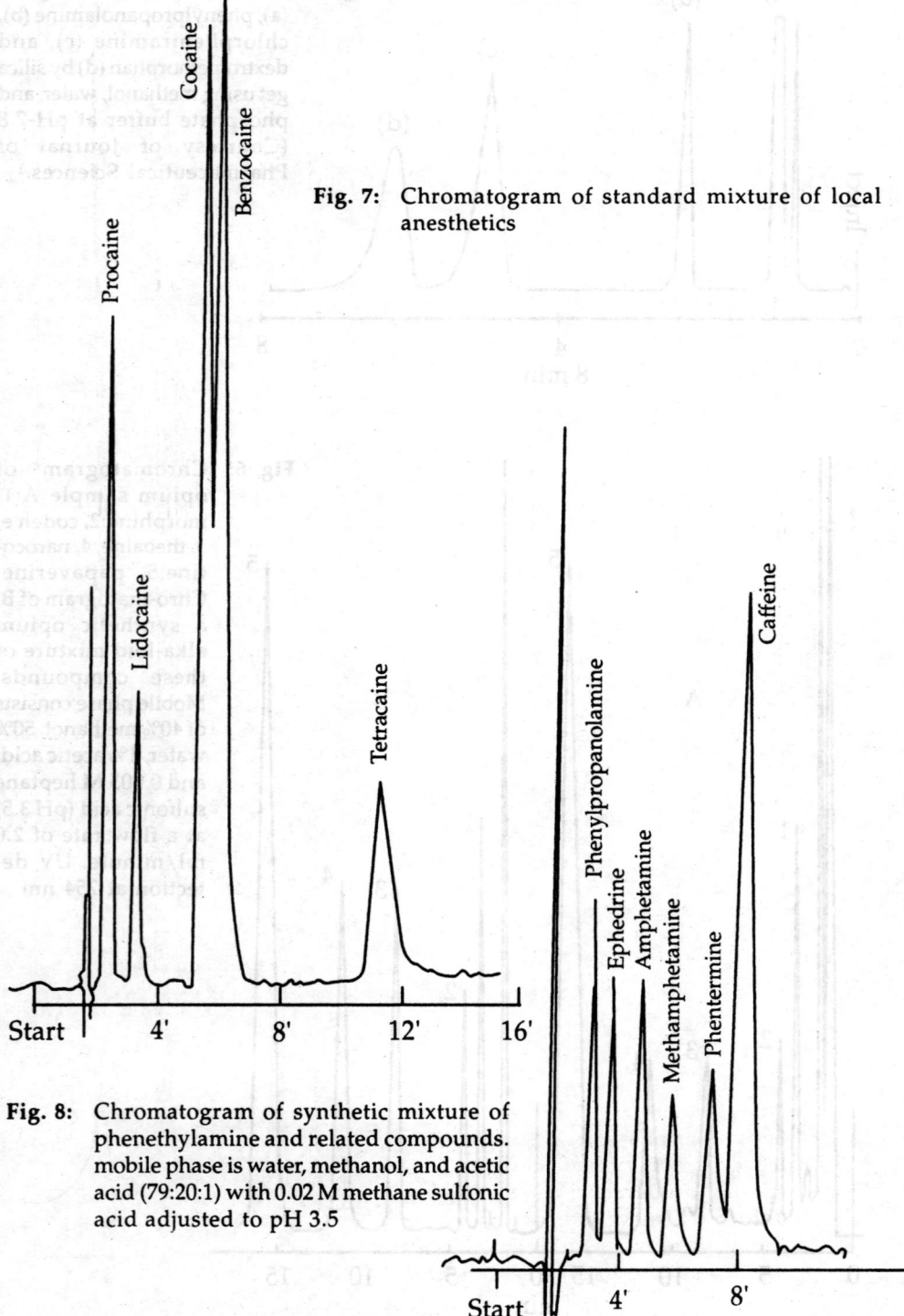

Fig. 7: Chromatogram of standard mixture of local anesthetics

Fig. 8: Chromatogram of synthetic mixture of phenethylamine and related compounds. mobile phase is water, methanol, and acetic acid (79:20:1) with 0.02 M methane sulfonic acid adjusted to pH 3.5

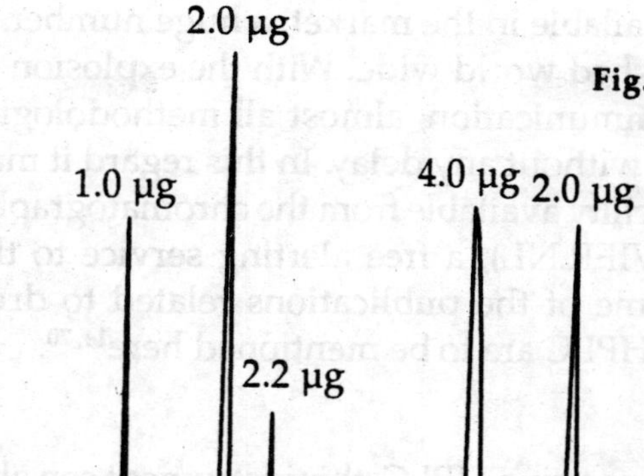

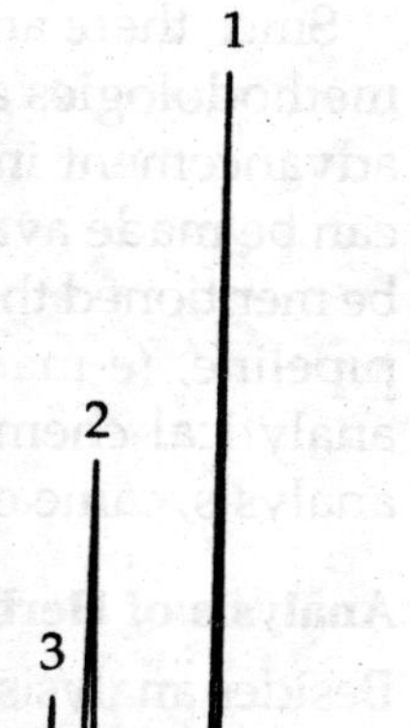

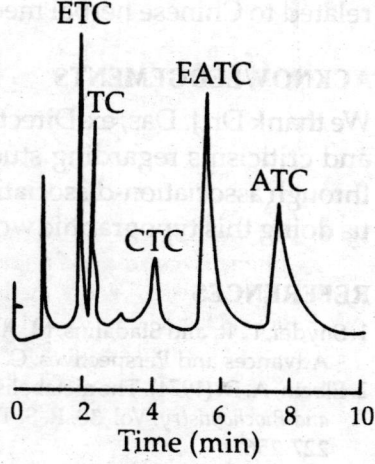

Fig. 10: Straight-phase separation of xanthine derivatives Column Lichrosorb Si60 5 im (300 × 3 mm ID), mobile phase dichloro-methane - etha-nol - water (936 : 47 : 17), flow rate 70 ml/h, detection UV 275 nm. Peaks: 1, caffeine, 2, theophylline; 3, thebromine

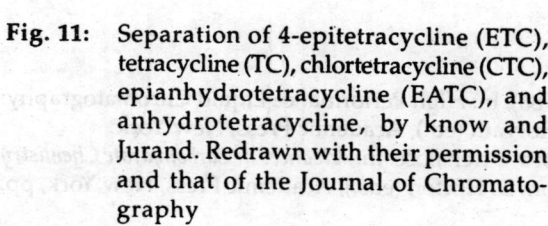

Fig. 9: HPLC of several penicillins

Fig. 11: Separation of 4-epitetracycline (ETC), tetracycline (TC), chlortetracycline (CTC), epianhydrotetracycline (EATC), and anhydrotetracycline, by know and Jurand. Redrawn with their permission and that of the Journal of Chromato-graphy

Since there are various drugs available in the market, a huge number of methodologies are regularly published world wide. With the explosion of advancement in the electronic communication, almost all methodologies can be made available to the users without any delay. In this regard it may be mentioned that there is a such facility available from the chromatography pipeline, (e-mail: A.AERT@ELSEVIER.NL), a free alerting service to the analytical chemists. Moreover, some of the publications related to drug analysis, came out recently, using HPLC are to be mentioned here[14, 20].

Analysis of Herbal Medicines

Besides analysis of conventional drug using HPLC, this instrument can also be a very powerful tool in a quality control laboratory attached to an industry manufacturing herbal medicines. Since exact chemical constituents present in a particular herbal product is mostly unknown, user should be very cautious before applying the sample into an expensive instrument like HPLC. General recommendation should be, first determine a condition in which all constituents present in the sample to be analysed remain completely soluble. Perhaps GP-HPLC is the first choice since there should be almost no interaction between the ingredients present in the sample and the stationary phase. It is also very important to determine the type of detector to be used for this kind of analysis. Perhaps a UV-detector, adjusted to very low wave length (200-220 nm) might be the first choice since almost all chemicals have absorbency in this range. Once all these are determined one must expect a characteristic chromatogram for a particular product. This should not vary from batch to batch or as a function of storage. Once an average chromatogram for a particular product is generated, this can be used as a reference during batch standardisation, etc. If a particular company is interested to proceed further, *e.g.*, identification of active ingredient(s), etc., other modes of HPLC may be attempted. In this regard, a recent work related to Chinese herbal medicine, may be mentioned[21].

ACKNOWLEDGEMENTS

We thank Dr. J. Das, ex-Director of this institute for his valuable suggestions and criticisms regarding studies related to regulation of protein function through association-dissociation. We also thank Mr. S. K. Chhatui for helping us doing this typographic work.

REFERENCES

1. Snyder, L. R. and Stadalius, M. A. (1986). In: High Performance Liquid Chromatography: Advances and Perspectives. C. S. Horvath (ed.), Academic Press, New York.
2. Elbein, A. D. (1974). The metabolism of a, a-trehalose. In: *Advances in Carbohydrate Chemistry and Biochemistry*, Vol. 30, R. S. Tipson, D. Horton (eds.), Academic Press, New York, pp. 227-256.

3. Werner-Washburne, M., Braun, E., Johnston, G. C. and Singer, R. A. (1993). Stationary phase in the yeast *Saccharomyces cerevisiae. Microbiol. Rev.,* **57**: 383-401.

4. Biswas, N. and Ghosh, A. K. (1997). Possible role of isoaspartyl methyltransferase towards the regulation of acid trehalase activity in *Saccharomyces cerevisiae. Biochim. Biophys. Acta,* 1335, 273-282.

5. Ghosh, A. K., Naskar, A. K. and Sengupta, S. (1997). Characterisation of xylanolytic amyloglucosidase of *Termitomyces clypeatus. Biochim. Biophys. Acta,* **1339**: 289-296.

6. Ghosh, A. K., Goswami, P. K. and Sengupta, S. (1992). Ion suppression chromatographic analysis of saturated lower fatty acids present during propionic acid fermentation. *J. Indian Chem. Soc.,* **69**: 572-573.

7. Baaij, J. A. D., Janssen, F. W. and Voortman, G. (1986). The use of an amino acid analyzer in food quality control. *Science Tools,* 33: 17-23.

8. Seipke, G., Mullner, H. and Grau, U. (1986). High-Pressure Liquid Chromatography (HPLC) of Proteins. *Angew. Chem. Int. Ed. Engl.,* **25**: 535-552.

9. Huang, J. X. and Guiochon, G. (1989). Applications of preparative high-performance liquid chromatography and purification of peptides and proteins. *J. Chromatogr.,* **492**: 431-469.

10. Regnier, F. E. (1987). The role of protein structure in chromatographic behaviour. *Science,* **235**: 319-323.

11. Roy, S. B., Ghosh, A. K., Sengupta, S. and Sengupta, S. (1994). Development of high-molar mass cellobiase complex by spontaneous protein-protein interaction in the culture filtrate of *Termitomyces clypeatus. Folia Microbiol.,* **39**: 463-470.

12. Biswas, N. and Ghosh, A. K. (1996) Characterisation of an acid trehalase of *Saccharomyces cerevisiae* present in trehalase-sucrose aggregate. *Biochim. Biophys. Acta,* **1290**: 95-100.

13. Biswas, N. and Ghosh, A. K. (1998). Regulation of acid trehalase activity by association-dissociation in Saccharomyces cerevisiae. *Biochim. Biophys. Acta,* **1379**: 245-2256.

14. Elliott, S. P. and Hale, K. A. (1997). Development of a high-performance liquid chromatographic retention index scale for toxicological drug screening. *J. Chromatogr. B: Bimed. Applications,* **694**: 99-114.

15. Chen, A. G., Wing, Y. K., Chiu, H., Lee, S., Chen, C. N. and Chan, K. (1997). Simultaneous determination of imipramine, desipramine and their 2- and 10-hydroxylated metabolites in human plasma and urine by high-performance liquid chromatography. *J. Chromatogr. B: Bimed. Applications,* **693**: 153-158.

16. Lopez-Calull, C., Gracia-Capdevila, L., Arroyo, C. and Bonal, J. (1997). Simple and robust high-performance liquid chromatographic method for the determination of ranitidine in microvolumes of human serum. *J. Chromatogr. B: Bimed. Applications,* **693**: 228-232.

17. Monaghan, J. M., Cook, K. G. D. and Crowther, D. (1997). Determination of nitrite and nitrate in human serum. *J. Chromatogr. A,* **770**: 143-149.

18. Everett, S. A., Dennis, M. F., Patel, K. B. Wardman, P. and Stratford, M. R. L. (1997). High-performance ion chromatography applied to free-radical mechanisms in drug design. The problem of ion analysis at high ionic strengths. *J. Chromatogr. A.,* **770**: 273-279.

19. Delbeke, F. T. and De Backer, P. (1996). Threshold level for theophylline in dopping analysis. *J. Chromatogr. B: Bimed. Applications,* **687**: 247-252.

20. Olsen, B. A. and Argentine, M. D. (1997). Investigation of response factor ruggedness for the determination of drug impurities by HPLC with ultraviolet detection L. *J. Chromatogr. A,* **762**: 227-233.

21. Chuan, L., Homma, M. and Oka, K. (1997). Chromatographic identification of phenolic compounds in human urine following oral administration of the herbal medicines Daisaiko-to and Shosaiko-to. *J. Chromatogr. B: Bimed. Applications,* **693**: 191-198.

6

MICRODIALYSIS AND ITS APPLICATION IN BIOAVAILABILITY STUDIES

H. Roustai* and A. K. Dash**

INTRODUCTION

The bioavailability of a drug is defined as "the rate and extent to which the active ingredient or active moiety is absorbed from a drug product and becomes available at the site of action. For drug products that are not intended to be absorbed into the bloodstream, bioavailability may be assessed by measurements intended to reflect the rate and extent to which the active ingredient or active moiety becomes available at the site of action" (Federal Register 2002). Bioavailability studies attempt to measure the relative fraction of the administered oral dose that is absorbed in the systemic circulation when compared to other dosage forms such as intravenous infusion (Federal Register 2002). With the advancement of targeted drug delivery, it is essential to determine the availability of the active moiety at or near the targeted tissue site rather than in the systemic circulation. Therefore, bioavailability studies can also be more precisely focused on a specific tissue to determine the drug distribution to the target site or organ. This chapter will focus on microdialysis as a sampling technique, which has recently become a very powerful tool in assessing tissue bioavailability.

Microdialysis is a sampling technique used both *in vivo* and *in vitro*. This technique has been utilized as early as 1966 by Bito and coworkers to determine the concentration of neurotransmitters in the central nervous system (CNS) in animals (Bito *et. al.*, 1966). Microdialysis involves the implantation of a probe into a tissue or to an *in vitro* medium. The probe consists of a semipermeable membrane continuously perfused at a definite rate with a physiological solution that is isotonic to the extracellular fluid. Depending on the molecular weight cut off of the membrane, low molecular weight compounds that are smaller than the pore size of the membrane can diffuse into or out of the probe lumen from a higher to a lower concentration. However, molecules larger than the pore size such as proteins and enzymes

*Department of Pharmacy Sciences, School of Pharmacy and Health Professions, Creighton University, Omaha, NE 68178, USA.
**Corresponding Author: Phone: (402) 280-3188, Fax: (402) 280-1883, Email: adash@creighton.edu

are excluded. The concentration of the molecules of interest in the perfusate is then monitored using a sensitive analytical method. Therefore, in case of microdialysis the driving force is based on a size-selective diffusion of an analyte between the tissue or medium surrounding the probe and the probe itself through the semipermeable membrane. At the outlet of the probe, the dialysate along with any endogenous substances (drugs or neurotransmitters) are collected. Microdialysis technique provides a continuous and clean sampling over a period of time.

In order to evaluate the bioavailability of an active moiety, a sensitive analytical method is required for the analysis of the drug in the systemic circulation. This includes radioisotopes, Immunoassays and chromatography with different detection modes such as ultraviolet, electrochemical, fluorescence and mass spectrometry. However, the chromatographic methods, which are extensively used for this purpose, require an additional sample preparation step to remove the protein from the sample prior to injection on to the HPLC column. Removal of protein is typically accomplished by protein precipitation, liquid extraction, solid-phase extraction or by supercritical fluid extraction methods. Additional sample preparation procedure in general results in a more complicated, laborious-multistep analysis scheme with an inherent decrease in precision and increase in assay time. Microdialysis sampling on the other hand offers several advantages for *in vivo* drug bioavailability studies. Since proteins are excluded from the sample by the dialysis membrane, the dialysate samples are protein-free and can be directly injected into the chromatographic system. Microdialysis allows real *in vivo* sampling from live, free moving animals over a prolonged period. It also allows determination of the concentration of the active moiety at a specific target organ or tissue. An elaborate review on the analytical considerations necessary for microdialysis sampling has been reported elsewhere (Davies *et. al.*, 2000).

The application of microdialysis in evaluating bioavailability of a drug can be broadly classified into two groups: (*i*) *in vitro* studies, and (*ii*) *in vivo* studies.

In Vitro Applications

In vitro dissolution testing of dosage forms is not a guarantee of therapeutic efficacy, but it is the best available in vitro method that can reveal qualitatively the physiological availability of a drug. According to the FDA Generic Drug Advisory Committee the dissolution testing is an in vitro surrogate marker for bioavailability and bioequivalence (AAPS Newsletter, 1994). Use of microdialysis in dissolution studies of drug was first reported in 1994 (Shah *et al.*, 1994). Authors in this study demonstrated the advantages of micro-dialysis sampling during in vitro dissolution studies. Advantages of this method include its versatility and easy automation, which allows use over a wide range of analyte concentrations, and in various dissolution media regardless of their pH. These authors in 1995 also documented the possible automation of multivessel dissolution testing system based on microdialysis sampling (Shah *et al.*, 1995). Knaub *et al.* studied the partitioning behavior of a fluoroquinolone across an erythrocyte *in vitro* using microdialysis (Knaub *et al.*, 1995). Dash and coworkers developed an *in vitro* dissolution method using microdialysis sampling technique for implantable drug delivery systems as shown in Fig. 1 (Dash, *et al.*, 1999). The advantages of this method include its simplicity and its requirement for a small volume of dissolution medium. In addition, it allows for online analysis, determination of drug concentration next to the implant, and provides continuous monitoring of the drug over a prolonged period.

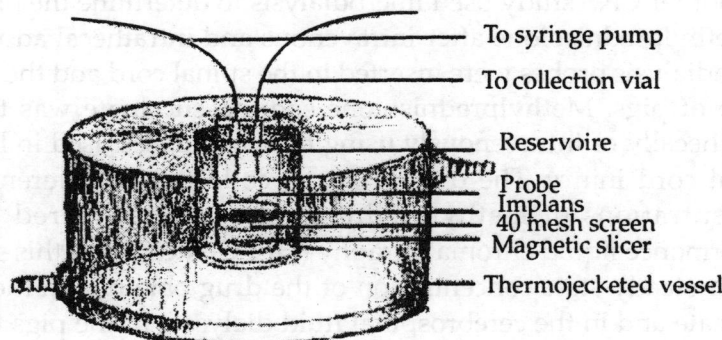

To syringe pump
To collection vial
Reservoire
Probe
Implans
40 mesh screen
Magnetic slicer
Thermojecketed vessel

Fig. 1: *In Vitro* dissolution apparatus for implantable drug delivery system. Reprinted from *J. Pharm. Sci.*, 88, Dash *et al.*, Development of in vitro dissolution method using microdialysis sampling technique for implantable drug delivery systems, 1036-1040, 1999 with permission.

In Vivo Applications

In vivo microdialysis has been extensively used to obtain information on drug distribution to clinically relevant target sites. A review in this effect has already been published elsewhere (Muller, 2000). Accessible tissues where microdialysis has been successfully used clinically include soft tissues (adipose and skeletal muscle), skin, CNS, neoplastic, heart, blood, lung and bone. Bioavailability evaluation using microdialysis sampling technique has been extensively studied in the CNS, eye, skin, and neoplastic tissue. The bioavailabilities of various drugs and pharmaceutical dosage forms have also been compared using microdialysis sampling technique. Some of the most relevant recent studies will be briefly reviewed below.

CNS Studies

A review on the use of microdialysis in CNS drug delivery has been published by Hammarlund-Ydenaes (Hammarlund-Ydenaes *et al.*, 2000). Another extensive review on the use of microdialysis to study the drug transporters in the CNS has also been published elsewhere (Sawchuk and Elmquist, 2000). CNS microdialyis experiments have accessed the bioavailability of various drugs and dosage forms to neural tissues and to the epidural space. Dexamethasone safety when delivered to the lumbar subarachnoid space was accessed in one experiment. In this study, rats received dexamethasone sodium phosphate either through a continuous injection intrathecally or via a bolus. In order to determine the bioavailability of dexamethasone sodium phosphate intrathecally, microdialysis was used to determine the kinetics of conversion of the prodrug dexamethasone sodium phosphate to the active drug dexamethasone (Kroin *et al.*, 2000).

Another CNS study used microdialysis to determine the bioavailability of methylprednisolone after intravenous and intrathecal administrations. Microdialysis probes were inserted in the spinal cord and the subarchnoid space of pigs. Methylprednisolone sodium succinate was then injected intrathecally or intravenously using the same doses used in humans with spinal cord injury. The dialysate was collected at different times. The concentrations of methylprednisolone were measured using high-performance liquid chromatography (HPLC). Results of this study show a higher steady state concentration of the drug obtained in the spinal cord dialysate and in the cerebrospinal fluid dialysate of the pigs that received intrathecal methylprednisolone as opposed to intravenous administration (Koszdin *et al.*, 2000).

Microdialysis sampling has been used to compare the bioavailability of different drugs and dosage forms. Clements *et al.* used microdialysis in two of their studies. In the first, microdialysis probe and catheters were inserted in the intrathecal or epidural spaces of rabbits to compare the bioavailability of bupivacaine and lidocaine (Clement *et al.*, 1999). Results of this study showed an increased cerebrospinal fluid (CSF) bioavailability of epidural bupivacaine as compared to lidocaine. The second study was conducted with both drugs administered at the same time (Clement *et al.*, 2000). Mode of administration and sampling methods used in this study are depicted in Fig. 2.

Results of the second study showed an increased intrathecal bioavailability of bupivacaine when the drug was co-administered intrathecally with lidocaine as compared to when it was administered alone. An increased mean CSF bioavailability of bupivacaine (12.3%) after simultaneous epidural administration with lidocaine was also observed as compared to when it was administered alone (5.5%).

The effect of lipid content of the liposomes and hydrophobicity of the drug on the epidural bioavailability of opiods has been reported by Bethune *et al.*, 2001. In this study, epidural and intrathecal spaces were continuously sampled via microdialysis. The rate of appearance of morphine and sufentanil in the epidural space of the pig was then determined. This study revealed that morphine was released more slowly than sulfentanil *in vivo*. In addition, increase in the lipid content in the morphine-loaded liposomes increased the proportion of drug released into the intrathecal space. However, increase in lipid content of the sulfentanil liposomes did not alter the intrathecal movement of this drug rather decreased its movement into plasma. Therefore, this study confirms that lipid content of the liposomes as well as hydrophobicity of the drug can affect the bioavailability of epidurally administered liposome encapsulated opioids in pigs.

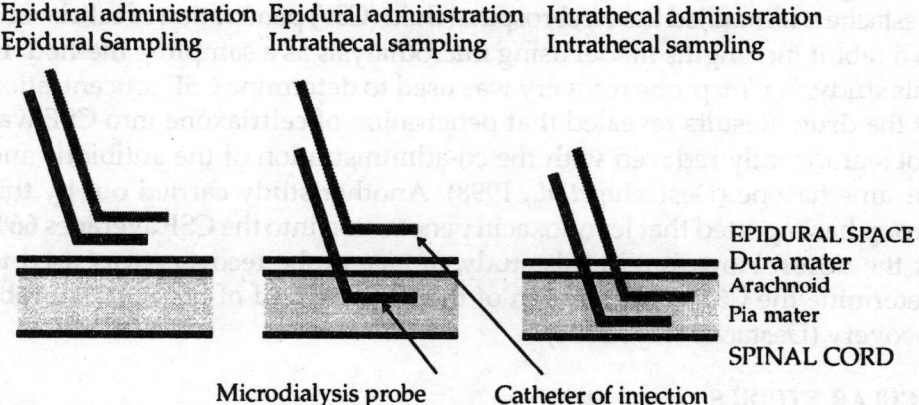

Epidural administration   Epidural administration   Intrathecal administration
Epidural Sampling   Intrathecal sampling   Intrathecal sampling

EPIDURAL SPACE
Dura mater
Arachnoid
Pia mater
SPINAL CORD

Microdialysis probe   Catheter of injection

Fig. 2: Schematic representation of the insertion of the microdialysis probe and of the catheter for drug administration. Reprinted from *Int. J. Pharm.*, 203, Clement *et al.*, Spinal biopharmaceutics of bupivacaine and lidocaine by microdialysis after their simultaneous administration in rabbits, 227-234, 2000 with permission.

Studies on the brain uptake of drug have also been reported using microdialysis sampling technique. One such study attempted to determine the effect of phenserine on acetylcholine level in rat brain (Greig *et al.*, 2000). A microdialysis probe was placed in the right corpus striatum of live rats and was fixed to the skull with dental cement. Dialysate samples were collected 24 hours later for the determination of mean basal acetylcholine levels in brain extracellular fluid by HPLC. Dialysate was then consecutively collected after phenserine administration. A time-dependant acetylcholine inhibition curve was obtained for the oral and intravenous administration of phenserine. Two other studies calculated the AUC from concentration versus time curves of endogenous neurotransmitters to determine the bioavailability of various drugs (Rodenhuis *et al.* 2000a and 2000b). One study compared the effect of series thiophene analogs including naphthxazines and 2-aminotetralins on dopamine levels in rat brains. Concentration versus time curves for dopamine was obtained by using brain microdialysis in freely moving animals. The relative bioavailability of the compound was obtained by comparing their AUC's to that of a standard compound 5-hydroxy-2-(N,N,-di-n-propylamino) tetralin (5-OH-DPAT). The introduction of thiophene moiety has shown to improve significantly the relative oral bioavailability as compared to 5-OH-DPAT. A similar study determined the oral bioavailability of R(-)apomorphine and its three analogs by comparing their AUC for dopamine release (Rodenhuis *et al.* 2000b). This study compared the ability of these three analogs in decreasing the release of dopamine in the striatum after subcutaneous and oral administration using microdialysis technique in freely moving rat. Two out of the three analogs investigated did not show any substantial improvement in bioavailability. Destache *et al.* studied the cerebrospinal fluid (CSF) penetration of ceftriaxone in a rabbit meningitis model using microdialysis as a sampling method. In this study, *in vitro* probe recovery was used to determine CSF concentration of the drug. Results revealed that penetration of ceftriaxone into CSF was not significantly reduced with the co-administration of the antibiotic and dexamethasone (Destache *et al.*, 1998). Another study carried out by this group has reported that levofloxacin penetration into the CSF averages 66% of the doses. However, in this study, *in vivo* probe recovery was used to determine the CSF concentration of the drug instead of the *in vitro* probe recovery (Destache *et al.*, 2001).

OCULAR STUDIES

Numerous studies on the bioavailability of various drugs in the vitreous humor and more recently in the ocular anterior segment have been carried out. Rittenhouse and Pollack have published a concise review on the use of microdialysis and the drug delivery to the eye (Rittenhouse and Pollack, 2000). The rabbit eye has been extensively used for this purpose. However, in some studies, cats, dogs and pigeons have been utilized. Using microdialysis sampling of aqueous humor, Rittenhouse *et al.* have reported that intraocular tissue availability of propranolol was significantly different in dogs as compared to rabbits (0.056 in case of dog and 0.55 in case of rabbit) (Rittenhouse *et al.*, 1996). Using microdialysis sampling in conscious rabbits, and in contrast to an earlier report, Rittenhouse and coworkers have shown that no saturable uptake of ascorbate from blood to aqueous humor was detected at a physiological concentrations of 11-30 mg/L (Rittenhouse *et al.*, 2000).

A major limitation to the study of ocular bioavailability of drugs is the inaccessibility of the vitreous humor. Intraocular pressure and variations in the formation of aqueous humor also impact the bioavailability studies of a drug in the eye (Rittenhouse and Pollack, 2000). A recent study attempted to develop a dual probe microdialysis technique for the simultaneous sampling of the vitreous and aqueous humor (Macha and Mitra, 2001a). In this study, two probes where inserted into the eye of rabbits. A linear probe was inserted in the aqueous humor and a concentric probe was implanted in the vitreous chamber as depicted in Fig. 3.

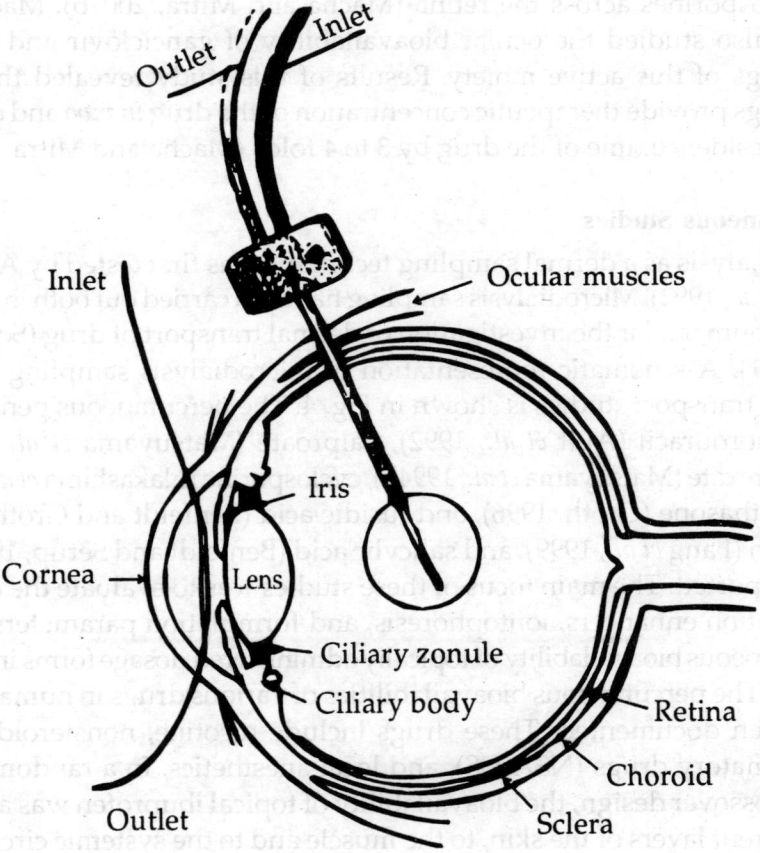

Fig. 3: Microdialysis probes used in evaluating ocular bioavailability of drugs. Reprinted from *Exp. Eye Res.*, **72**, Macha and Mitra, Ocular pharmacokinetics in rabbits using a novel dual probe microdialysis technique, 289-299, 2001a with permission.

Next, the aqueous and vitreous elimination kinetics of fluorescein was studied after intravitreal and systemic administration into the marginal ear vein. Microdialysis samples were collected every 20 minutes over a period of 10 hours. A concentration versus time profile was then obtained and the rate of elimination of the drug was calculated. In a similar study, the same authors determined the ocular pharmacokinetics of cephalosporins in rabbits (Macha and Mitra, 2001b). A concentric microdialysis probe was implanted in the vitreous chamber and a linear probe was inserted across the cornea in the aqueous humor similarly to the previous experiment. Isotonic phosphate buffer saline was perfused through the probes, and samples were collected every 20 min over a period of 10 hr. The vitreal half-lives of cephalexin, cefazolin, and cephalothin were determined and compared. This study demonstrated the involvement of peptide carrier in the transport of cephalosporines across the retina (Macha and Mitra, 2001b). Macha and Mitra also studied the ocular bioavailability of ganciclovir and various prodrugs of this active moiety. Results of this study revealed that ester prodrugs provide therapeutic concentration of the drug *in vivo* and enhance mean residence time of the drug by 3 to 4 folds (Macha and Mitra, 2002).

Percutaneous Studies

Microdialysis as a dermal sampling technique was first tested by Ault *et al.* (Ault *et al.*, 1992). Microdialysis sampling has been carried out both in animals and in humans for the investigation of dermal transport of drug (Schnetz *et al.*, 2001). A schematic representation of microdialysis sampling used in dermal transport studies is shown in Fig. 4. The percutaneous penetration of 5-fluorouracil (Ault *et al.*, 1992), valproate (Matsuyama *et al.*, 1994a), methotrexate (Matsuyama *et al.*, 1994b), cyclosporine (Nakashima *et al.*, 1996), betamethasone (Groth, 1996), and fusidic acid (Benfeldt and Groth, 1998), Enoxain (Fang *et al.*, 1999), and salicylic acid (Benfeldt and Serup, 1999) has been reported. The main focus of these studies was to evaluate the effect of penetration enhancers, iontophoresis, and formulation parameters on the percutaneous bioavailability of topically administered dosage forms in animal model. The percutaneous bioavailabilities of various drugs in humans have also been documented. These drugs include nicotine, nonsteroidal anti-inflammatory drugs (NSAIDS), and local anesthetics. In a randomized 2-way crossover design, the bioavailability of topical ibuprofen was assessed to different layers of the skin, to the muscle and to the systemic circulation. Subjects in this study received either two 400-mg ibuprofen tablets or 16 g of a 5% ibuprofen gel.

Dialysate was then collected every 20 minutes over a period of 5 hours. Urine metabolite concentrations were analyzed with HPLC. The relative bioavailability of the gel to that of the oral administration was determined by comparing the ratio of the total amount of ibuprofen excreted in 24 hours. Results of this study indicated that dialysate concentration was increased consistently with plasma concentrations when the drug was given orally. However, after cutaneous administration a very high variability in dialysate concentrations among the patients were seen in both the muscle and the skin possibly due to inter-individual differences in the stratum corneum.

Results also indicated that cutaneous drug concentration was higher after topical administration as compared to oral administration. This study demonstrates that inter-patient variability in drug absorption through the skin is one of the major challenges one has to take into account during transcutaneous drug delivery system development.

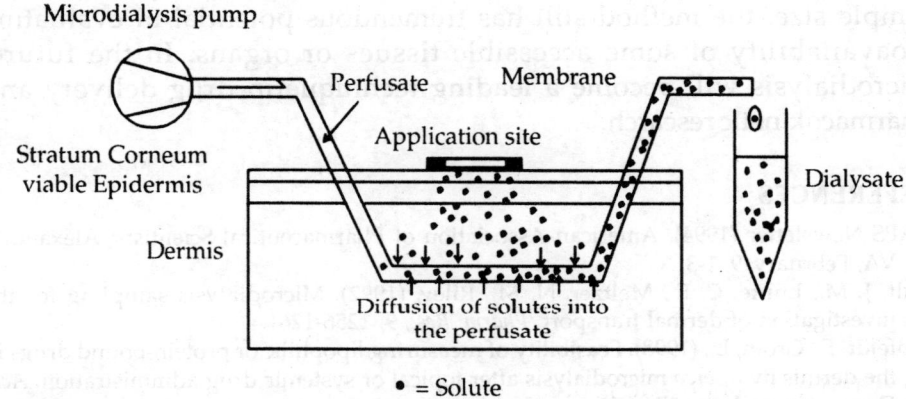

Fig. 4: Schematic representation of a dermal microdialysis sampling. Reprinted from *Eur. J. Pharm. Sci.*, **12**, Schnetz and Fartassch, Microdialysis for the evaluation of penetration through the human skin barrier-a promising tool for future research, 165-174, 2001 with permission.

Blood and Other Tissues

Microdialysis has recently been used for the measurement of free drug in the blood circulation in humans (O'Connell *et al.*, 1996, Patsalos, *et al.*, 1996, Paez *et al.*, 1997). This technique is advantageous in blood bioavailabiliy studies since samples are free from endogenous protein and only concentration of the free drug is determined. In addition, if the drug is not stable in the plasma or blood, it can be stabilized after collection into the sampling tube. Blood microdialysis studies are achieved by placing special types of flexible and robust probes in the arteries or veins. Dizdar *et al.* have studied the L-dopa concentration in healthy as well as in patients with Parkinson disease. Intravenous and subcutaneous microdialysis was performed to compare the free concentration of L-dopa in blood and compared with data obtained with ordinary venous blood sampling (Dizdar, *et al.*, 1999). Results of this study suggest that L-dopa has a 50% protein binding and is rapidly distributed to various tissues. Microdialysis has also been used to determine the bioavailability of amoxicillin in the middle ear fluid in awake chinchilla (Huang *et al.*, 2001). Microdialysis and its application in oncology research and treatment are gaining tremendous momentum. Microdialysis allows direct study of the tumor drug exposure and metabolism in a minimally invasive way (Brunner and Muller, 2002).

CONCLUSION

Microdialysis has provided scientist new opportunities to study the bioavailability and distribution of drug at specific tissue sites. This article covers the application of this vastly growing technique in assessing the tissue bioavailability of various drugs and drug delivery systems. Although this method does have some limitations, such as the ability to only assess small sample size, the method still has tremendous potential in evaluating bioavailability of some accessible tissues or organs. In the future, microdialysis will become a leading technique in drug delivery and pharmacokinetic research.

REFERENCES

AAPS Newsletter (1994). American Association of Pharmaceutical Scientists: Alexandria VA, February. 9, 1-3.

Ault, J. M., Lunte, C. E., Meltzer, N. M., Riley, (1992). Microdialysis sampling for the investigation of dermal transport. *Pharm. Res.*, **9**: 1256-1261.

Benfeldt, E., Groth, L., (1998). Feasibility of measuring lipophilic or protein-bound drugs in the dermis by *in vivo* microdialysis after topical or systemic drug administration. *Acta Derm. -Venereol.* **78**: 274-278.

Benfeldt, E., Serup, J., (1999). Effect of barrier perturbation on cutaneous penetration of salicylic acid in hairless rats: *in vivo* pharmacokinetics using microdialysis and non-invasive quantification of barrier function. *Arch. Dermatol. Res.*, **291**: 517-526.

Bethune, C. R., Bernards, C. M., Bui-Nguyen, T., Shen, D. D., Ho, R. J. Y., (2001). The role of drug-lipid interactions on the disposition of liposome-formulated Opioid analgesics and *in vivo*. *Anesth. Analg.*, **93**: 928-933.

Bito, L., Davson H., Levin E., Murray M., Snider, N., (1966). The concentrations of free aminoacids and other electrolytes in cerebrospinal fluid, *in vivo* dialysate of brain, and blood plasma of the dog. *J. Neurochem.*, **13**: 1057-1067.

Brunner, M., Muller, M., (2002). Microdialysis: an *in vivo* approach for measuring drug delivery in oncology. *Eur. J. Clin. Pharmacol.*, **58**: 227-234.

Clement, R., Malinovsky, J. M., Corre, P. L., Dollo, G., Chevanne, F., Verge, R. L., (1999). Cerebrospinal fluid bioavailability and pharmacokinetics of bupivacaine and lidocaine after intrathecal and epidural administrations in rabbits using microdialysis. *J. Pharm.-Exp.-Ther.*, **289**: 1015-1021.

Clement, R., Malinovsky, J. M., Corre, P. L., Dollo, G., Chevanne, F., Verge, R. L., (2000). Spinal biopharmaceutics of bupivacaine and lidocaine by microdialysis after their simultaneous administration in rabbits. *Int. J. Pharm.*, **203**: 227-234.

Dash, A. K., Haney, P. W., Garavalia, M C., (1999). Development of *in vitro* dissolution method using microdialysis sampling technique for implantable drug delivery systems. *J. Pharm. Sci.*, **88**: 1036-1040.

Davies, M. I., Cooper, J. D., Desmond, S. S., Lunte, C. E, Lunte, S. M., (2000). Analytical considerations for microdialysis sampling. *Adv. Drug Deliv. Rev.*, **45**: 169-88.

Destache, C. J., Pakiz, C. B., Dash, A. K., Larsen, C., (1998). Nitric oxide concentration and cerebrospinal fluid parameters in an experimental animal model of *Streptococcus pneumoniae meningitis*. *Pharmacotherapy*, **18**: 612-619.

Destache, C. J., Pakiz, C. B., Larsen, C., Owens, H. and Dash, A. K., (2001). Cerebrospinal fluid penetration and pharmacokinetics of levofloxacin in an experimental rabbit meningitis model. *J. Antimicrob. Chemo.*, **47**: 611-615.

Didzar, N., Kullman, A., Norlander, B., Olsson, J. E., Kagedal, B. (1999). Human pharmacokinetics of L-3, 4-dihydroxyphenylalanine studied with microdialysis. *Clin. Chem.*, **45**: 1813-1820.

Fang, J. Y., Hsu, L. R., Huang, Y. B., Tsai, Y. H., (1999). Evaluation of transdermal iontophoresis of enoxain from polymer formulations: in vitro skin permeation and in vivo microdialysis using wistar rat as animal model. *Int. J. Pharm.*, **180**: 137-149.

Federal Register, (2002). Guidance for Inaustry: Bioavailability and bioequivalence studies for orally administered drug products—General consideration. Draft Guidance, Federal Register, 2002, p. 3.

Greig, N. H., Micheli, E. D., Hollwoway, H. W., Yu, Q. S., Utsuki, T., Perry, T. A., Brossi, A., Ingram, D. K., Deutsch, J., Lahiri, D. K. and Soncrant, T. T. (2000). The experimental Alzheimer drug phenserine preclinical pharmacokinetics and pharmacodynamics. *Acta Neurol. Scand.*, **176(S)**: 74-84.

Groth, L. (1996). Cutaneous microdialysis, methodology and validation. *Acta Derm. Venereol.*, **76(S)**: 197.

Knaub, S. R., Chang, M. F., Lunte C. E., Topp E. M., Riley, C. M., (1995). Automated analytical systems for drug development studies. Part IV. A microdialysis system to study the parttioning of lomefloxacin across an erythrocyte membrane *in vitro. J. Pharm. Biomed. Anal.*, **14**: 121-129.

Koszdin, K. L., Shen, D. D., Bernards, C. M., (2000). Spinal cord bioavailability of methylprednisolone after intravenous and intrathecal administration: The role of P-glycoprotein. *Anethesiology*, **92**: 156-163.

Kroin, J. S., Schaefer, R. B., Penn, R. D. (2000). Chronic intrathecal administration of dexamehasone sodium phosphate: pharmacokinetics and neurotoxicity in an animal model. *Neurosurgery*, **46**: 178-183.

Macha, S., Mitra, A. (2001a). Ocular pharmacokinetics in rabbits using a novel dual probe microdialysis technique. *Exp. Eye Res.*, **72**: 289-299.

Macha, S., Mitra, A. (2001b). Ocular pharmacokinetics of cephalosporins using microdialysis. *J. Ocul. Pharmacol. Ther.*, **17**: 485-498.

Macha, S., Mitra, A. (2002). Ocular disposition of ganciclovir and its monoester prodrugs following intravitreal administration using. *Drug Metab. Dispos.*, **30**: 670-675.

Matsuyma, K. Nakashima, M., Ichikawa, M., Yano, T., Satoh, S., Goto, S. (1994a). In vivo microdialysis for the transdermal absorption of valproate in rats. *Biol. Pharm. Bull.* **17**: 395-398.

Matsuyma, K. Nakashima, M., Nakaboh, Y., Ichikawa, M., Yano, T., Satoh, S. (1994b). Application of *in vivo* microdialysis to transdermal absorption of methotrexate in rats. *Pharm. Res.*, **11**: 684-686.

Muller, M. (2000). Microdialysis in clinical drug delivery studies. *Adv. Drug Del. Rev.*, **45**: 255-269.

Nakashima, M., Zhao, M. F., Ohya, H., Sakurai, M., Sasaki, H., Matsuyama, K., Ichikawa, M. (1996). Evaluation of in vivo transdermal absorption of cyclosporin with absorption enhancer using intradermal microdialysis in rats. *J. Pharm. Pharmcol.*, **48**: 1143-1146.

O'connell, M. T., Tison, F., Quinn, N, Patsalos, P. (1996). Clinical drug monitoring by microdialysis: application to levodopa therapy in Parkinson's disease. *Br. J. Pharmacol.*, **42**: 765-769.

Patasalos, P. N., O'connell, M. T., Doheny, H. C., Sander, JWAS, Sharvon, S. D. (1996). Antiepileptic drug pharmacokinetics in patients with epilepsy using a new microdialysis probe: preliminary observations. *Actr Neurochir. Suppl.*, **67**: 59-62.

Paez, X. Hernadez, L. (1997). Blood microdialysis in humans: a new method for monitoring plasma compounds. *Life Sci.*, **61**: 847-856.

Rittenhouse, K. D., Peiffer, R. L., Pollack, G. M. (1996). Evaluation of microdialysis sampling of aqueous humor for in vivo models of ocular absorption and disposition. *J. Pharm. Biomed. Anal.*, **16**: 951-959.

Rittenhouse, K. D., Peiffer, R. L., Pollack, G. M. (2000). Assessment of ascorbate ocular disposition in the conscious rabbit: an approach using the microdialysis technique. *Curr. Eye Res. Anal.*, **20**: 351-360.

Rittenhouse, K., Pollack, G. M. (2000). Microdialysis and drug delivery to the eye. *Adv. Drug Del. Rev.*, **45**: 229-241.

Rodenhuis, N., Dijkstra, D., Boer, P., Vermeulen, E. S., Timmerman, W., Wikstrom, H. V., (2000a). Dopamine D2activity of R-(-)-apomorphine and selected analogs: a microdialysis study. *Eur. J. Pharmacol.*, **387**: 39-45.

Rodenhuis, N., Timmerman, W., Wikstrom, H. V., Dijkstra, D. (2000b). Thiophene analogs of naphthoxazines and 2-aminotetralins: bioisosteres with improved relative oral bioavailability, as compared to 5-OH-DPAT. *Eur. J. Pharmacol.*, **394**: 255-263.

Sawchuk, R. J., Elmquist, W. F. (2000). Microdialysis in the study of drug transporters in the CNS. *Adv. Drug Del. Rev.*, **45**: 295-307.

Schnetz, E., Fartasch, M. (2001). Microdialysis for the evaluation of penetration through the human skin barrier-a promising tool for future research. *Eur. J. Pharm. Sci.*, **12**: 165-174.

Shah, K. P., Chang M., Riley, C. M., 1995. Automated analytical systems for drug development studies. III. Multivessel dissolution testing system based on microdialysis sampling. *J. Pharm. Biomed. Anal.*, **13**: 1235-1241.

Shah, K. P., Chang, M., Riley, C. M., (1994). Automated analytical systems for drug development studies. II. A system for dissolution testing. *J. Pharm. Biomed. Anal.*, **12**: 1519-1527.

Tegeder, I., Selbach, U. M., Lotsch, J., Rusing, G., Oelkers, R., Brune, K., Meller, S., Kelm, G.R., Sorgel, F., Geisslinger, G. (1999). Application of microdialysis for the determination of muscle and subcutaneous tissue concentrations after oral and topical ibuprofen administration. *Clin. Pharmacol. Ther.*, **65**: 357-368.

7

OCULAR KINETICS AND DRUG DELIVERY SYSTEMS OF OPHTHALMIC MEDICINES— A REVIEW

Nihar R Biswas*, Alok K Ravi*, Tirlok C Chawla*

INTRODUCTION

Bioavailability may be defined more precisely as the rate and extent of absorption of a drug from its dosage into the systemic circulation. Bioavailability of a drug may be influenced by its rate of dissolution, disintegration or actual content of the drug. Formulation factor may significantly modify the onset, intensity and duration of therapeutic response, the incidence and intensity of side effects and the stability of the product.[1]

The overall absorption rate constant of a drug is the net effect of two processes occurring simultaneously, the dissolution of the drug in fluids at the absorption site and the passage of dissolved drug across the membrane at the absorption site.[2] Change in pharmaceutical preparation of one brand of a drug may show different intrinsic absorption pattern from other.

Clinical observations have confirmed enormous differences in the activity of a drug administered in the same dosage from different manufacturers.[3] Schneller[3] reported on 40 different drug substances with proven or suspected bioavailability problem. The overwhelming evidence makes it clear that chemical equivalence alone will not guarantee biological or therapeutic equivalence.[3]

OCULAR DRUG THERAPY

Topical drug therapy is preferred in all sight threatening conditions like endophthalmitis, corneal ulcers, trachoma and glaucoma etc., to maintain adequate drug levels in the ocular tissues. Eye drops are easily administered and may be immediately active, but the medication stays on the eye surface for very short time. Applying ointments and suspensions prolong the stay of the drug on the eye surface, which facilitates absorption, but they cause inconvenience due to poor vision, increased viscosity and stickiness. Intravitreal and sub-conjunctival injections are other forms of drug therapy, which are only preferred in emergency conditions. Insoluble or soluble ocular

*Dr. Rajendra Prasad Centre for Ophthalmic Sciences, AIIMS, New Delhi-110 029.

inserts constitute an improved drug delivery system but their usage is limited due to their poor-availability and exorbitant price.[4] Patients often have difficulty in placing and retaining a solid insert in the cul-de-sac and also suffer from foreign body sensation evoked by these devices.[4] Other alternative approaches like oral administration of drug or parenteral administration fail to achieve optimum concentration at the required site due to the presence of ocular-blood barrier.[5]

The potential clinical utility of a drug is assessed by the amount of active ingredient(s) delivered and maintained at its site of action when applied to the eye. Ocular structures posing protective mechanisms for the eye allow only 1% or even less than that of the instilled dose of the drug to actually reach the anterior segment tissues of the eye.[5] Further, only a fraction of the absorbed dose penetrates to posterior tissues from the most frequently used dosage forms *i.e.* ophthalmic solutions, ointments and other forms of medications.[6] Drugs are further compromised in their effectiveness by limitations like poor penetration through the lipophilic corneal barrier, non-productive absorption through the conjunctiva and rapid nasolacrimal drainage.[5] Moreover, corneal penetration of water-soluble drugs is poor as compared to lipid-soluble drugs.[5] To overcome these shortcomings, there is an inevitable need for newer drug delivery systems.

Ocular Absorption

An ophthalmic medicine must be available to the part of the eye that is intended to and it must be available in sufficient concentrations to have the desired effect. Some drugs, such as contact lens solutions, eyewashes and irrigating solutions, are required to reach only to the tear film, whereas other drug must pass into the conjunctiva or through the cornea to carry out their intended actions.[7] Most drugs must be compatible with the physical chemistry of the tears, the cornea, and the conjunctiva.

Systemic Absorption

It may seem unlikely that the small quantities of the ophthalmic drugs generally applied topically could be absorbed systemically in sufficient amounts to cause any systemic effect. Numerous case reports and laboratory studies indicate however, that topically applied drugs are absorbed systemically in some cases with profound effect.[8]

DRUG INTERACTIONS WITH TEARS

Many ophthalmic preparations are developed to affect only on external surface of the eye. It is therefore necessary that these solutions be able to mix evenly with the tears and remain in the lacrimal sac sufficiently long to produce their intended effect. These pharmaceuticals include contact lens wetting agents, artificial tears, and antibiotic drugs to treat conjunctivitis or blepharitis.[6] When a water-soluble drug is applied to the eye, it mixes rapidly with the tears. The conjunctival sac normally holds about 7 μl of fluid. When a person is not allowed to blink, it can temporarily hold about 25 μl.[9] One drop from a standard eyedropper contains about 30-50ul of fluid; thus, the majority of the drop that is applied is immediately lost by flowing either over the lid margin or down the nasolacrimal duct. Another cause of rapid drug loss from the external eye is the constant turnover of tears as new tears are secreted, flow over the eye, and are lost down the nasolacrimal duct.[9] Estimation of the tear turnover rate varies between 0.66-1.2 μl / min.[10] Due to tear dilution, the concentrations of the drug in the tears remain about 50 percent in the first minute and within 8 minutes to about 1/1000th of its initial concentration.[11]

As the concentration of the drug falls, the diffusion gradient forcing it into the eye is also reduced. As the tears dilute the drug, more is lost through normal tear drainage; thus, a large proportion of the drug does not remain in the eye.[12] For example, after application of 0.1 ml of a 2 % solution of radioactive pilocarpine in rabbits, the peak intraocular concentration was measured after 15 minutes, but even at that time, less than 1 % of the instilled drug could be found in any ocular structures.[5] The total amount absorbed depends upon the particular drug used.

DRUG INTERACTIONS WITH THE CORNEA

If a drug is to act on an internal ocular structure such as the iris, it must be able to penetrate the cornea. Only cornea is responsible to penetrate the drug into the eye. This was shown by applying disks soaked with radioactive compound either to the conjunctiva or to the cornea.[5, 13] A substantially higher concentration of radioactive drug could be found in ocular tissues when the disks were applied to the cornea than when they were applied to the conjunctiva.[5, 13] An understanding of the characteristics of the cornea is therefore necessary to predict whether a drug will enter the eye readily.

DRUG INTERACTIONS WITH THE CONJUNCTIVA

After intraocular surgery, steroids may be injected subconjunctivally to act as a reservoir of the drug.[14] Most of the drug does not enter the eye directly from the reservoir through the sclera. It is believed that most of the drug that enters the eye first flows out from depot into the tears, and then through the cornea, and into the eye.[14] However, considerable systemic absorption may occur through the conjunctival blood vessels in case of hyperemic conjunctiva.

OCULAR KINETICS

Ocular kinetics is the science that deals with absorption, distribution, metabolism and excretion of a drug(s) in the eye. Therapeutic becomes more rational when it follows the principles of ocular pharmacokinetics.

When a drug is introduced into the human body, it diffuses through various cell membranes and binds to proteins in the blood or tissues.[15] Such processes occur at various rates and to varying extent, depending upon the physico-chemical characteristics of the drug. Consequently, a given drug should produce a specific plasma time-distribution pattern reflected by the measured drug concentrations in the plasma.[2]

It is assumed that drugs are uniformly distributed in the body. When we consider the body as a single compartment within which, a drug appears to be uniformly distributed then we can assume that the concentrations of the drug in the plasma or blood to be the same as in all other tissues.[1] Since the concentration of drug in the various parts of the body may be quite different, the volume of the compartment derived from the concentration of a drug in plasma or blood does not necessarily reflect a real body fluid volume and, therefore, is called apparent volume of distribution.[1]

The apparent volume of distribution (V) is proportional to the body weight (wt.)

$$V = v^1 \text{ wt.} \quad \text{(where } v^1 = \text{coefficient of distribution)}$$

The ocular pharmacokinetic parameters like absorption, apparent volume of distribution and elimination rate constant of phenylephrine and the prodrug were determined from aqueous humor concentration-time and mydriasis-time profiles by Chein et al in 1990.[16] The study showed that the kinetic parameters of phenylephrine estimated from its mydriasis profile do not accurately reflect the kinetics of drug distribution in the iris.[16] These parameters also varied with the instillation of phenylephrine solution or prodrug suspensions.[16] A mydriatic tolerance of the pupil response was apparent after the topical instillation of phenylephrine solutions. It was conducted from the study that reduction in mydriatic tolerance may be due to the decrease in number of receptors on the iris dilator muscles.[16]

Topical treatment of severe ocular infections might require the use of fortified antibiotic in concentration beyond commercially available preparations.[17] The authors studied tear pharmacokinetics, tissue bioavailability, epithelial toxicity, and compared with antibacterial efficacy of topical tobramycin of 0.3-5 % concentrations. Tear pharmacodynamics study showed that the bioassay-measurable levels are higher with each preparation up to 6 hours after a single 50 µl drop. Comparing of various fortified concentration levels yielded progressive parallel-biphasic decay curves in antibiotic tear concentrations.[17] Both tear and corneal data demonstrated increase in antibiotic levels largely proportional to the increase in drug concentrations instilled. A *Pseudomonas aeruginosa* keratitis model in the rat demonstrated the antibiotic efficacy of topical tobramycin treatment over untreated controls ($p < 0.00001$), and a progressively enhanced efficacy with increasing tobramycin concentrations is suggested.[17] It was concluded from the study that concentration enhancement of topical ocular medications are useful in the treatment of severe ocular infections.[18]

Classical pharmacokinetic theory based on the studies of systemically administered drugs does not fully apply to all ophthalmic drugs. Although, similar principles of absorption, distribution, metabolism, and excretion determine the fate of drug disposition in the eye, ophthalmic medications are applied topically using a variety of formulations. Drugs also may be injected by subconjunctival, sub-tenons, and retrobulbar routes. For example, anaesthetic agents are administered commonly by injection for surgical procedures. 5-fluorouracil, an anti-metabolite and anti-proliferative agent may be administered subconjunctivally to retard the fibroblast proliferation related to scarring after glaucoma surgery.[19] Intraocular injections of antimicrobial agents are considered in the treatment of endophthalmitis. The sensitivities of the organisms to the antibiotic and the retinal toxicity threshold may be nearly the same for some antibiotics; hence, the antibiotic dose, injected intravitreally must be carefully titrated.[20]

Unlike clinical pharmacokinetic studies on systemic drugs, where data are collected relatively easily from blood samples, there is significant risk in obtaining tissue and fluid samples from the human eye.[21] Consequently, animal models are studied to provide pharmacokinetic data on ophthalmic drugs. Commonly, the rabbit is used for such studies.

OCULAR DRUG DELIVERY SYSTEMS

Topical drug treatment of ocular diseases has the difficulty of achieving a sufficient quantity of drug at the desired site of action. For ocular drugs, to be effective an ideal drug delivery system (DDS) should provide the drug at the receptor site of the ocular tissues in relatively higher concentrations to elicit the desired pharmacological response. The tight junctions of iris capillaries and retina act as a barrier to the diffusion of drugs from the blood into the aqueous and vitreous and the cornea acts as a barrier to drugs applied topically.[5]

Most important factor, which modifies drug penetration, is slow release of the drug, thereby increasing the contact time of the drug to the ocular tissues.[4] The duration of the drug action in the eye can be extended by (*i*) improving corneal drug penetration (*ii*) reducing drainage through the use of viscosity enhancing agents.[22] Factors that affect the bioavailability of ocular drugs include pH, salt form of the drug,[23] vehicle composition, osmolality, toxicity and viscosity.

Kanpolat *et al.* 24 used commercially available 12 hours collagen shields to deliver cyclosporin A (CsA) to the cornea and aqueous humour in the rabbit eyes. In their study, six New Zealand white rabbits were divided into three groups. The first group (4 eyes) received 6 mg of CsA in castor oil and the second group (4 eyes) received 6 mg of CsA in olive oil applied as topical drops to rabbit eyes within 12 hours. In the third group (4 eyes) 12 hours collagen shields soaked in 6 mg CsA in olive oil were applied to the rabbit eyes. The results of their study showed that the CsA levels of castor oil drops were higher than those obtained with olive oil drops. In eyes with collagen shields, CsA levels were higher than olive oil drops but nearly equal to the castor oil drops. Collagen shields may be useful as an ocular drug delivery system for cyclosporin A.

The most frequently used ocular therapeutics are eye drops, ointments and inserts. Independence on the physico-chemical properties of the therapeutical substance and the kind of disease, one has to formulate the form of the drug in the manner to obtain its maximal bioavailability. By increasing their viscosity one can keep the watery solutions in the conjunctival sac for around 60 minutes.[6] The time of contact of the drug, given in the form of suspension is limited mainly by the viscosity of the solution and the size of the molecules suspended in it.[25] The ointments stay on the surface of the eye up to 2 hours.[26] The ocular inserts secure a steady flow of the therapeutical substance up to 7 days.[7] The compounds penetrate into the anterior chamber of eye mainly through the cornea. Therefore the physiological factors of the lacrimal fluid, the properties of the cornea may influence the penetration of the corneo-chamber barrier by the therapeutical substance.[25]

Chiang *et al.* studied in rabbits, two timolol preparations, a gel and an eyedrop of thickening agent, and one commercial eyedrops without a thickening agent.[27] After topical administration of these three preparations in rabbit eyes, aqueous humor withdrawn and the proteins removed from the samples by precipitation with acetonitrile. Timolol concentrations determined directly by the HPLC method. Methanol and d-camphorsulfonic acid (in 1% acetic acid) in a ratio of 49 : 51 (v/v) used as HPLC mobile phase. A reversed phase C-18 column used to separate samples with a flow rate of 0.8 ml/min and a UV detector set at 284 nm. A two-compartment pharmacokinetic model was used to fit the aqueous humor level for determining the drainage (kd) and absorption rate constants (ka) in the precorneal area as well as the elimination rate constant (ke) of timolol in aqueous humor. For ka + kd, the eyedrop without a thickening agent had the highest value (0.160 per minute), followed by the eyedrop with a thickening agent (0.030 per minute), and the gel had the lowest value (0.009 per minute). It suggested that the gel has a longer retention time in eyes to improve ocular bioavailability and decrease side effects.

Carbomer based hydrogel with timolol maleate (T-Gel) used for the study as a vehicle effect on ocular bioavailability.[28] Pharmacokinetic profiles of T-Gel 0.05% (0.05% timolol), T-Gel 0.025% (0.025% timolol) and commercial timolol ophthalmic solution (TOS 0.1%; 0.1% timolol) determined and compared. Timolol detected in the washings up to 1 hr after instillation of test products; the highest levels observed after T-Gel 0.05%. Their study concluded that the new vehicle obviously improves the bioavailability of topically applied timolol.

Burgalassi *et al.* [29] in their study aimed at verifying the performances of a mucoadhesive polysaccharide from tamarind seed [Xyloglucan or tamarin seed polysaccharide (TSP)], as an adjuvant for ophthalmic vehicles containing timolol. Three formulations (one experimental vehicle based on TSP and the reference commercially eye drops) containing 5 mg/ml timolol base equivalents were administered to the eyes of pigmented rabbits. Drug concentrations in tear fluid, cornea, iris-ciliary body, aqueous humor and plasma were determined, as well as intraocular pressure was measured.

The polymer under investigation, in spite of a comparatively low viscosity, produced high performances of the TSP vehicle were comparable to those of a reference "*in situ*" gelling formulation (Timoptic XE). The results pointed to TSP as a potentially useful adjuvant for ophthalmic delivery systems.

MEDICATION FORMS USED IN OPHTHALMOLOGY
Solutions, Ointments, Sprays, Gels, Lid scrubs.

Solutions
Most of the topical ocular preparations are commonly available as solutions which are applied directly to the eye. Eye drops is one of the most common forms of drug delivery systems. A "Pouch method of eye drop instillation" has been described[7] whereby the patient looks up and the lower eyelid is held averted. The eye drop is placed into the exposed lower cul-de-sac and allowed to pool there. The eyelids are then gently closed and kept closed for 2-5 minutes so that blinking does not activate the lacrimal pump system.

Ointments
Clinically significant enhancement of drug penetration results from the prolonged contact time with eye. Ointments are especially useful for treating children who may not co-operate for topically applied solutions. Ointments are especially useful for medicating ocular injuries such as corneal abrasions

where the eye needs to be patched. A practical problem with ointment instillation is the difficulty of delivering a small volume of medication. The ribbon of ointment cannot be easily separated from the tubing without contacting the eye, which contaminates the tube. The commonly used ophthalmic ointment bases and liquid oily vehicles are made up of lanolin, petrolatum and peanut oil, which are toxic to the interior of the eye, causing endothelial damage, corneal oedema, vascularization, and scarring.[26, 30] For this reason, ophthalmic medications in ointment or oily liquid vehicles should not be instilled into the interior of the eye. Experimental studies showed that introduction of 0.1 ml of any of these substances into rabbit eyes caused severe reactions with secondary glaucoma.

Sprays

This form is specially used for pediatric patients and solution is administered using a sterile perfume atomizer or plastic spray bottle. Mydriatics-cycloplegics can be administered as spray to the closed eye to dilate the pupil.[31]

Gels

Corticosteroids dispensed in gel vehicles may contain therapeutic levels 5 times or more longer than in ordinary liquid vehicles. Ophthalmic gels are similar in viscosity and clinical usage to ophthalmic ointments. Experimental trials indicate that delivery of pilocarpine in viscous gel vehicles instilled twice daily may control intraocular pressure as well as solutions of equal drug strength instilled 4 times daily.

Lid Scrubs

Eyelid cleansers, antibiotic solutions or ointments can be applied directly to the eyelid margin for the treatment of blepharitis. This is ideally achieved by applying the medicationtipped applicator and then scrubbing the eyelid margins several times daily.

DRUG DELIVERY DEVICES IN OPHTHALMOLOGY

- O Ocusert System
- O Drug Impregnated Inserts—Soluble Ophthalmic Drug Inserts [SODI]
- O Hydrogel contact lens
- O Corneal collagen shields
- O Filter paper strips
- O Cotton pledgets

○ Lacriserts (Artificial tear inserts)
○ Continuous irrigation
○ Nanoparticles
○ Gel-forming erodible inserts
○ Micro-emulsions

Ocusert System

The Ocusert is a device with a two-membrane sandwich with a pilocarpine reservoir in the centre. The co-polymeric membrane is ethylene vinylacetate with a pilocarpine reservoir in the centre. A white titanium dioxide ring incorporated between the membrane that helps in visualizing and handling the inserts.[7] Ocuserts are soft and extremely flexible and can be placed either under the upper or lower lid. Ocuserts provide a zero-order rate of delivery by steady-state diffusing whereby drug is released at a more constant rate to the pre-corneal tear film over a finite period of time rather than as a bolus.[32]

Although membrane controlled drug delivery has advantages and is effective in some patients, the inserts have not gained widespread use, likely due to their cost and the fact that patients often have difficulty placing and retaining a solid insert in the cul-de-sac. Drugs that can be delivered through Ocusert are pilocarpine, antibiotics, steroids and carbachol.

Drug Impregnated Inserts

Soluble ocular drug inserts (SODI) are made of polymers of ethylacrylate, vinyl pyrolidone and acrylamide. SODI dissolve in cul-de-sac and is capable to provide detectable drug levels in the cornea upto 48 hours. Wafers are inserts made of succinylated collagen. Wafers are 6 mm × 12 mm in size and are inserted into the inferior cul-de-sac.[4]

In the treatment of keratoconjunctivitis sicca, a 12 mg cellulosic polymer rod is itself the active ingredient. The rod is supplied sterile, without preservative. When inserted in the lower cul-de-sac in the morning, the substance slowly dissolves during the day and stabilizes the tear film. A particular advantage of this method is that no preservative is necessary. Thiomersol and chlorbutanol may be toxic to the dry eye. Benzalkonium chloride, a detergent, de-stabilizes the tear film.

Hydrogel Contact Lens

Higher water content with large intermolecular pore size contact lens has the capability to absorb water-soluble drugs and release gradually.[33] Dexamethasone, antibiotics and pilocarpine can be delivered through hydrogel contact lens.[34] Maximum drug delivery is obtained by presoaking the lens. The permeability of drug is related to thickness of the lens. A thinner lens allows a greater amount of topically applied drug to pass into the lens-cornea interface. It is used in the treatment of dry eye syndromes and in bullous keratopathy. Jain [35] compared soft contact lens delivery with subconjunctival delivery of chloramphenicol, gentamicin and carbenicillin. Soft contact lenses give significantly higher aqueous drug levels than subconjunctival injection.

Collagen Corneal Shields

Collagen shields have been studied extensively for their potential usefulness as drug delivery devices because the drug is released as the shield dissolves.[36] Collagen shields are made of thin membranes of porcine or bovine scleral collagen.[37] Collagen shields are packaged in a dehydrated state and require rehydration before application, when a shield is rehydrated in a solution containing a water-soluble drug, the drug becomes trapped in the collagen matrix, shields dissolve as a result of proteolytic degradation by the tear film.[37] Use of collagen shields in conjunction with topical trifluridine has been found to shorten the average epithelial healing time of herpes simplex keratitis compared with traditional antiviral eye drop therapy.[38] Clinical experience indicates that the collagen shield is relatively safe when used as a drug delivery device. Drug delivery using impregnated collagen shields is potentially more comfortable and reliable than frequent applications of eye drops or subconjunctival injections.[39] Collagen shields are superior to topical eyedrops or soft contact lenses in delivering water-soluble drugs to the human cornea.[40] Following are the limitations to use collagen shields.

- O Highest cost
- O Limited number of base curves and diameters
- O Shields degrade over a short time
- O Drug precipitation occurs if drug combination used.
- O Corneal hypoxia with tight lens syndrome.

Filter Paper Strips

Sodium fluorescein, rose bengal and lissamine green are commercially available as drug impregnated filter paper strips. Fluorescein impregnated paper strips eliminates the risk of solution contamination with *Pseudomonas aeruginosa*. For administration, the drug-impregnated paper strip moistened with a drop of normal saline, and the applicator is gently touched to the superior or inferior bulbar conjunctiva or to the inferior conjunctival sac.

Cotton Pledgets

A pledget is constructed by simply teasing the cotton tip of an applicator to form a small (5mm) elongated body of cotton. These devices allow prolonged ocular time with solutions that are normally topically instilled into the eye. After placing one or two drops of the ophthalmic solution on the pledget, the device is placed into the inferior conjunctival fornix. This device of drug delivery allows maximum mydriasis in attempts to break posterior synechiae or dilate sluggish pupils.

Lacrisert (artificial tear inserts)

It consists of a rod shaped pellet of hydroxy propyl cellulose without preservative. Each lacrisert is 1 mm in diameter and 4 mm in length at dehydrated state and it contains 5 mg of the synthetic polymer. Lacrisert is inserted into the inferior conjunctival fornix. After placement into the conjunctival sac, its hypertonicity causes it to absorb basal tear production and fluid from the capillaries of the conjunctiva, and swells, becoming a gelatinous mass. After several hours, the insert dissolves and releases the polymer into the tear film. Once-a-day application is usually sufficient to relieve symptoms. This device is useful for the patients with moderate to severe dry eye syndrome. Blurring of vision and foreign body sensations are two significant problems for user.[41] In patients with insufficient remaining basal tear secretion, the inserts do not imbibe fluid, dissolve, or release polymer to the eye and treatment may be failure with this device.[42]

Continuous Flow Devices

Conventional irrigating system-Extraocular irrigation is used to dislodge foreign material in the initial treatment of acute chemical burns and ocular foreign bodies. It consists of the container of irrigating solution and a tissue paper or towel with which to collect the fluid after bathing the eye. Patients should be in a supine position with head tilted toward the side to be irrigated with the upper and lower lids retracted; the clinician gently bathes the extra ocular surfaces with the solution. *Continuous irrigating system*—Most methods that have been devised for continuous ocular irrigation are suitable for short periods in non-ambulatory patients. Polyethylene tubing is sometimes simply passed with a minor surgical procedure through the lid and into the conjunctival fornix, and the fluid or drug to be perfused is supplied from an overhead infusion bottle. The tubing is anchored to the skin with sutures and may also be secured by tape. In cases in which it is undesirable to penetrate the lids surgically, various configurations of tubing, loops, rings and haptic contact lens shells have been successfully used.[43] The Morgan lens is the convenient commercially available system. This system is capable of delivering a continuous flow of saline to every surface of the eye and conjunctival sac. Fluid flow, acts as a cushion and allow the lens to float above the cornea and below the eyelid, avoiding contact with damaged ocular tissues.

Nanoparticles

Some specific drugs are recognised by molecules that are involved in the disease. These drugs are then able to act directly on their relevant targets. For other diseases, like inflammatory diseases and cancer, drug molecules are much less specific, and considerable side effects are seen with these drugs. If we could deliver these drugs to a specific location, the disease could be treated more effectively with reduced side effects.

To overcome this problem, drugs are incorporated into small particles, which could release their drug at the site of interest. It has been found that the particles need to be very small, around 50-150 nm in diameter to reach suitable targets.[44] Also that the particles need to be coated to make them invisible to the body's immune system to avoid them being prematurely removed by organs like the cornea and liver. The best coatings to use are very hydrophilic molecules such as polyethylene glycol (PEG), which do not interact with these defence receptors.[45] The nanoparticles are produced by an instantaneous self-assembly process and are micellar in nature with the poly lactide (PLA) segments forming the core of the particle and the PEG segments forming a mobile corona. The PLA core is solid, and the density of the PEG corona varied as the block sizes of the PLA and the PEG are changed. Investigations are done with both biodegradable particles with adsorbed surface layers and micellar type particles made by phase separation techniques from block copolymers of poly (lactide)-poly (ethyleneglycol) (PLA-PEG).[46] The resulting polymers are used to make nanoparticles which were characterised by a variety of physicochemical techniques including: transmission electron microscopy (morphology),[47] Infrared (IR) spectroscopy (hydrodynamic diameter),[48] NMR (structure of particles in D_2O),[49] hydrophobic interaction chromatography, colloidal stability in salt solutions. The biological performance of nanoparticles is believed to derive from the adsorption of specific serum proteins to the PEG layer. Following three drugs are under development for nanoparticle delivery applications— Conventional low molecular weight drugs, protein and polypeptide drugs, and DNA for oligonucleotide or gene therapy.

Gel-forming Erodible Inserts[50]

A new ocular drug delivery of high molecular weight (400 KDa) linear poly (ethylene oxide) (PEO) in gel-forming erodible inserts for ocular controlled application of ofloxacin (OFX) has been tested in vitro and in vivo. Inserts of 6 mm diameter, 20mg weight and soaked with 0.3 mg OFX, were prepared by powder compression. The in vitro drug release from inserts was mainly controlled by insert erosion. The rate of insert erosion depended on the strength of inter-polymer interactions in the compounds, and on the hydrophilic balance of compounds. Compared to commercial OFX eyedrops, drug absorption into the aqueous humor was retarded by the PEO-EUDNa 71% inserts (Poly(ethylene oxide)-Eudragit L100 71% Neutralised), and both retarded and prolonged by the PEO-EUDNa 17% inserts. $C_{(max)}$, $AUC_{(eff)}$ were strikingly increased by plain PEO inserts with respect to commercial eye drops.

Micro-emulsions[51]

The mechanism of micro-emulsions is based on the absorption of the nanodroplets representing the internal phase of the micro-emulsion, which constitutes a reservoir for the drug on the cornea.

The micro-emulsions are a promising dosage form for the natural defence of the eye because they are prepared by inexpensive processes through autoemulsification. They can be easily sterilized; they are stable and have a high capacity of dissolving the ocular drug. The *in vivo* results and preliminary studies on healthy volunteers have shown a delayed effect and an increase in the bioavailability of ophthalmic drug.

REFERENCES

1. Hardman, J. G. and Limbird, L. E. (2001). *Pharmacokinetics: The Dynamics of Drug Absorption, Distribution, and Elimination; The Pharmacological Basis of Therapeutics*, 10th ed, McGraw-Hill, New York.
2. Rowland, M., Tozer, T. N. (eds.) (1995). *Clinical Pharmacokinetics: Concepts and Applications*, 3rd ed. William & Wilkins, Philadelphia.
3. Schneller, G. H. (1969). Hazard of therapeutic nonequivalency of drug products. *J. Am. Pharm. Assoc.*, 9(9): 455-459.
4. Bourlais, C. L., Acar, L., Zia, H. *et al.* (1998). Ophthalmic drug delivery systems—recent advances. *Prog. Retin. Eye Res.*, 17: 33-58.
5. Harris, J. E. (1968). Problems in drug Penetration. In: Symposium on Ocular Therapy. St. Louis: C V Mosby, 3: pp. 96-106.
6. MacKeen, D. L. (1980). Aqueous formulations and ointments. *Int. Ophthalmol. Clin.*, 20(3): 79-92.
7. Bartlett, J. D., Jaanus, D. S. (2001). *Ophthalmic Drug Delivery: In Clinical Ocular Pharmacology* 4th ed. Butterworth Heinemann, New York.
8. Shell, J. W. (1982). Pharmacokinetics of topically applied ophthalmic drugs. *Surv. Ophthal.* 26(4): 207-218.
9. Fraunfelder, F. T. (1976). Extraocular fluid dynamics: how best to apply topical ocular medication. *Trans. Am. Ophthal. Soc.* 74: 457-487.
10. Patton, T. F. and Robinson, J. R. (1975). Influence of topical anesthesia on tear dynamics and ocular drug bioavailability in albino rabbits. *J. Pharm Sci.*, 64(2): 267-271.

11. Linn, M. L. and Jones, L. T. (1968). Rate of lacrimal excretion of ophthalmic vehicles. *Am. J. Ophthalmol.*, **65**(1): 76-78.

12. Mishima, S., Gasset, A., Klyce, S. D. Jr. and Baum, J. L. (1966). Determination of tear volume and tear flow. *Invest. Ophthalmol.* **5**(3): 264-275.

13. McCartney, H. J., Drysdale, I. O., Gornall, A. G. *et al.* (1965). An autoradiographic study of the penetration of subconjunctivally injected hydrocortisone into the normal and inflamed rabbit eye. *Invest. Ophthalmol.*, **4**(3): 297-302.

14. Wine, N. A., Gornall, A. G. and Basu, P. K. (1964). The ocular uptake of subconjunctivally injected C14 hydrocortisone. I. Time and major route of penetration in a normal eye. *Am. J. Ophthalmol.* **58**(3): 362-366.

15. Pratts, W. B., Taylor, P. (eds.) (1990). *Principles of Drug Action: The Basis of Pharmacology*, 3rd ed. Churchill Living Stone, New York.

16. Chien, D. S. and Schoenwald, R. D. (1990). Ocular Pharmacokinetics and pharmacodynamics of phenylephrine and phenylephrine oxazolidine in rabbit eyes. *Pharm. Res.* **7**(5): 476-483.

17. Gilbert, M. L., Wilhelmus, K. R. and Osato, M. S. (1987). Comparative bioavailability and efficacy of fortified topical tobramycin. *Invest. Ophthalmol. Vis. Sci.*, **28**(5): 881-885.

18. Chen, C. C., Takruri, H. and Duzman, E. (1993). Enhancement of the ocular bioavailability of topical tobramycin with use of a collagen shield. *J. Cataract Refract. Surg.*, **19**(2): 242-245.

19. Azuara, B. A., Moster, M. R. and Marr, B. P. (1997). Subconjunctival versus peribulbar anesthesia in trabeculectomy: a prospective, randomized study. *Ophthalmic. Surg. Lasers*, **28**: 896-899.

20. Peyman, G. A. and Schulman, J. A. (1989). Intravitreal drug therapy. *Jpn. J. Ophthalmol.*, **33**: 392-404.

21. Akers, M. J. (1983). Ocular bioavailability of topically applied ophthalmic drugs. *Am. Pharm.*, **23**(1): 33-36.

22. Putterman, A. M. (1985). Instilling ocular ointments without blurred vision. *Arch. Ophthalmol.*, **103**: 1276.

23. Osato, M. S. (1999). Effect of two balanced salt solutions on the bioavailability of ofloxacin and ciprofloxacin. *Adv. Ther.*, **55**(6): 440-443.

24. Kanpolat, A., Batioglu, F., Yilmaz, M. and Akbas, F. (1994). Penetration of cyclosporin A into the rabbit cornea and aqueous humor after topical drop and collagen shield administration. *CLAOJ*, **20**(2): 119-12?.

25. Zimmerman, T. J., Kooner, K. S., Kandarakis, A. S. *et al.* (1984). Improving the therapeutic index of topically applied ocular drugs. *Arch. Ophthalmol*, **102**(4): 551-552.

26. Hanna, C., Fraunfelder, F.T. and Cable, M., *et al.* (1973). The effect of ophthalmic ointments on corneal wound healing. *Am. J. Ophthalmol.*, **76**(2): 193-200.

27. Chiang, C. H., Ho, J. I. and Chen, J. L. (1996). Pharmacokinetics and intraocular pressure lowering effect of timolol preparations in rabbit eyes. *J. Ocul. Pharmacol. Ther.* Winter; **12**(4): 471-480.

28. Von der Ohe N., Stark, M., Mayer, H. and Brewitt, H. (1996). How can the bioavailability of timolol be enhanced? A pharmacokinetic pilot study of novel hydrogels. *Graefes Arch. Clin. Exp. Ophthalmol.*, **234**(7): 452-456.

29. Burgalassi, S., Chetoni, P., Panichi, L., Boldrini, E. and Saettone, M. F. (2000). Xyloglucan as a novel vehicle for timolol: pharmacokinetics and pressure lowering activity in rabbits. *J. Ocul. Pharmacol. Ther.*, **16**(6): 497-509.

30. Heerema, J. E. and Friedenwald, J. S. (1950). Retardation of wound healing in the corneal epithelium by lanalin. *Am. J. Ophthalmol.*, **33**(9): 1421-1427.

31. Bartlett, J. D., Wesson, M. D., Swiatocha, J. and Woolley, T. (1993). Efficacy of a pediatric cycloplegic administered as a spray. *J. Am. Optom. Assoc.*, **64**: 617-621.
32. Lamberts, D. W. (1980). Solid delivery devices. *Int. Ophthalmol. Clin.*, **20**(3): 63-77.
33. Aquavella, J. V. (1976). New aspects of contact lenses in ophthalmology. *Adv. Ophthalmol.*, **32**: 2-34.
34. Waltman, S. R., Kaufman, H. E. (1970). Use of hydrophilic contact lenses to increase ocular penetration of topical drugs. *Invest. Ophthalmol. Vis. Sci.*, **9**(4): 250-255.
35. Jain, M. R. (1988). Drug delivery through soft contact lenses. *Br. J. Ophthalmol.* **72**: 150-154.
36. Friedberg, M. L., Pleyer, U. and Mondino, J. (1991). Device drug delivery to the eye. Collagen shields, iontophoresis and pumps. *Ophthalmology*, **98**: 725-732.
37. Mondino, B. J. (1991). Collagen shields. *Am. J. Ophthalmol.*, **112**: 587-590.
38. Kuster, P., Travella, M., Gelinas, M. and Stepp, P. (1998). Delivery of trifluridine to human cornea and aqueous using collagen shields. *CLAOJ*, **24**: 122-124.
39. Taravella, M., Stepp, P., Young, D. (1998). Collagen shield delivery of tobramycin to the human eye. *CLAOJ*, **24**: 166-168.
40. Weissman, B. A., Brennan, N. A., Lee, D. A. and Fatt, I. (1990). Oxygen permeability of collagen shields. *Invest. Ophthalmol. Vis. Sci.*, **31**: 334-338.
41. Lindahl, G., Calissendorf, B. and Carle, B. (1988). Clinical trial of sustained-release artificial tears in keratoconjunctivitis sicca and sjögren's syndrome. *Acta. Ophthalmol.*, **66**: 9-14.
42. LaMotte, J., Grossman, E. and Herscn, J. (1985). The efficacy of cellulosic-ophthalmic inserts for treatment of dry eye. *J. Am. Optom. Assoc.*, **56**(4): 298-302.
43. Yamabayashi, S., Furuya, T., Gohd, T., *et al.* (1990). Newly designed continuous corneal irrigation system for chemical burns. *Ophthalmologica.*, **201**: 174-179.
44. Kreuter, J. (1983). *Pharm. Acta. Helv.*, **58**: 196-208.
45. Alonso, M. J. (2001). Polymeric nanoparticles: New system for improving ocular bioavailability of drugs. *Arch. Soc. Esp. Ophthalmol.*, **76**(8): 453-454.
46. Lipscomb, W. N., Jacobson, R. A. (1972). In: *Techniques of Chemistry*, III, Vol 1A. Weissberger and BW Rossiter (eds.) New York, Wiley-Inter Science.
47. Rollot, J. M., Schwarz, A., Rohdewald, P. *et al.* (1986). *J. Pharm. Sci.*, **75**: 361-364.
48. Lee Smith (1979). *Applied Infrared Spectroscopy: Fundamentals, Techniques and Analytical Problems Solving.* John Wiley & Sons, NY, Ch-5: pp. 186-194.
49. Abraham, R. J., Fisher, J., Loftus, P. (1988). *Introduction to Nuclear Magnetic Resonance Spectroscopy.* Wiley, New York.
50. Di Colo, G., Burgalassi, S., Chetoni, P., *et al.* (2001). Gel firming erodible inserts for ocular controlled delivery of ofloxacin. *Int. J. Pharm.*, **14**: 215 (1-2) 101-111.
51. Vandamme, T. F. (2002). Microemulsions as ocular drug delivery systems: recent developments and future challenges. *Prog. Retin. Eye Res.*, **21**(1): 15-34.

8

BIOEQUIVALENCE STUDY AND DATA INTERPRETATION

T. K. Pal* and M. Ganesan**

INTRODUCTION

The U.S. Food and Drug Administration define bioavailability as "the rate and extent to which the active ingredient or active moiety is absorbed from a drug product and becomes available at the site of action. Since pharmacologic response is generally related to the concentration of drug at the receptor site, the availability of a drug from a dosage form is a critical element of a drug product's clinical efficacy. For drug products that are not intended to be absorbed into the bloodstream, bioavailability may be assessed by measurements intended to reflect the rate and extent to which the active ingredient or moiety becomes available at the site of action". In practice it is difficult to determine the drug concentrations at the site of action. Therefore, bioavailability is more commonly defined as "the rate and extent of absorption of parent drugs or active metabolites from a dosage form into the systemic circulation."

Most bioavailability studies involve the determination of drug concentration in the blood or urine. This is based on the premise that the drug at the site of action is in equilibrium with drug in the blood. It is therefore possible to obtain an indirect measure of drug response by monitoring drug levels in the blood or urine. Thus, bioavailability is concerned with how quickly and how much of a drug appears in the blood after a specific dose is administered. The bioavailability of a drug product often determines the therapeutic efficacy of that product since it affects the onset, intensity and duration of therapeutic response of the drug. In most cases one is concerned with the extent of absorption of drug, (that is, the fraction of the dose that actually reaches the bloodstream) since this represents the "effective dose" of a drug. This is generally less than the amount of drug actually administered in the dosage form. In some cases, notably those where acute conditions are being treated, one is also concerned with the rate of absorption of a drug, since rapid onset of pharmacologic action is desired.

*Prof. Bioequivalence Study Centre, Department of Pharmaceutical Technology, Jadavpur University, Kolkata-32.

**Department of Pharmaceutical Technology, Jadavpur University, Kolkata-32.

Conversely, there are instances where a slower rate of absorption is desired, either to avoid adverse effects or to produce a prolonged duration of action.

"Absolute" bioavailability, F, is the fraction of an administered dose which actually reaches the systemic circulation, and ranges from F = 0 (no drug absorption) to F = 1 (complete drug absorption). Since the total amount of drug reaching the systemic circulation is directly proportional to the area under the plasma drug concentration as a function of time curve (AUC), F is determined by comparing the respective AUCs of the test product and the same dose of drug administered intravenously. The intravenous route is the reference standard since the dose is, by definition, completely available.

$$F = \frac{AUC_{ev}}{AUC_{iv}}$$

where AUC_{ev} and AUC_{iv} are, respectively, the area under the plasma concentration-time curve following the extravascular and intravenous administration of a given dose of drug. Knowledge of F is needed to determine an appropriate oral dose of a drug relative to an IV dose.

"Relative" or "Comparative" bioavailability refers to the availability of a drug product as compared to another dosage form or product of the same drug given in the same dose. These measurements determine the effects of formulation differences on drug absorption. The relative bioavailability of product A compared to product B, both products containing the same dose of the same drug, is obtained by comparing their respective AUCs.

$$Relative\ bioavailability = \frac{AUC_A}{AUC_B}$$

where drug product B is the reference standard. When the bioavailability of a generic product is considered, it is usually the relative bioavailability that is referred to. A more general form of the equation results from considering the possibility of different doses,

$$Comparative\ Bioavailability = \frac{\dfrac{AUC_{Generic}}{Dose_{Generic}}}{\dfrac{AUC_{Brand}}{Dose_{Brand}}}$$

To exert an optimal pharmacotherapeutic action, an active substance should be delivered at the site of its action in an effective concentration during the desired period. To allow prediction of the therapeutic effect, the performance of the pharmaceutical form containing the active substance should be reproducible. Several therapeutic misadventures in the past (digoxin, phenytoin, primidone) testify the necessity of this reproducibility as a quality requirement. Thus the bioavailability of an active substance from a pharmaceutical product should be known and be reproducible. This is especially the case if one product is substituted for another. In that case the product should show the same therapeutic effect in the clinical situation. It is generally cumbersome to assess this by clinical studies. Assuming that in the same subject an essentially similar plasma concentration time course will result in essentially similar concentrations at the site of action and thus in an essentially similar effect, pharmacokinetic data instead of therapeutic results may be used to establish equivalence: bioequivalence.

Bioequivalence or comparative bioavailability gained increasing attention during the last three decades after it became evident that marketed products having same amounts of drug chemical entity may exhibit marked differences between their therapeutic responses. In many instances, these differences were correlated successfully to dissimilar drug blood levels caused mainly by impaired absorption.

The availability of different formulations of the same drug substance given at the same strength and in the same dosage form poses a special challenge to health care professionals, making these issues very relevant to pharmacists in all practice settings. Since pharmacists play an important role in product-selection decisions, they must have an understanding of the principles and concepts of bioavailability and bioequivalence.

Bioequivalence is a relative term which indicates that the drug substances in two or more similar dosage forms reaches the systemic circulation at the same relative rate and to the same relative extent. In other words, the blood level profiles following administration of the two dosage forms are within an expected statistical variance, superimposable. Two medicinal products are bioequivalents if their bioavailabilities (rate and extent) after administration in the same molar dose are similar to such degree that their effects, with respect to both efficacy and safety, will be essentially the same.

In other words two products containing equal doses of a drug will be said to be bioequivalent if they do not differ significantly in either their bioavailable dose or its rate of supply[1]. Since the concentration of a drug in blood is used as an assessment of its clinical performance, inherent in the demonstration that two preparations containing equivalent amounts of the same drug produce similar concentrations of the drug entity in blood is the assumption that they will elicit equivalent drug responses. Thus, two products that are deemed to be bioequivalent are also assumed to be therapeutically equivalent, and therefore interchangeable. This principle is fundamental to the concept of bioequivalence and is the basic premise on which it is founded.

Variations in the bioavailability of drug products have been recognized as responsible for a few therapeutic failures. One example of therapeutic failure arising from variations in the bioavailability of ostensibly equivalent products involved the important and highly potent cardiotonic drug, digoxin. A number of patients were observed to require unusually large maintenance doses of digoxin despite the absence of any condition that might have explained a high tolerance to the drug. Upon investigation, the patients were found to have low digoxin concentrations in their blood plasma. A crossover study revealed striking differences in bioavailability among four digoxin preparations available in the same hospital at the time. The peak concentration after a single dose was found to vary among the four drug products by a factor of as much as seven. It is noteworthy that the margin of safety of this drug is sufficiently narrow that serious or even lethal toxic effects can result if the dose given and absorbed is as little as twice that needed to achieve a therapeutic effect.

Although there is a spectrum of opinion about the frequency and importance of differences in the bioavailability of chemically equivalent drug products, there can be no dispute about the fact that well-documented and significant differences in bioavailability have been demonstrated in chemically equivalent products representing a number of drug categories.

Problems of bioequivalence have received serious investigative attention only during the past few years. In this brief period, however, a number of studies of marketed drug products containing the same therapeutic ingredient have revealed marked differences in the rate and extent of absorption. A considerable body of literature has accumulated in this period that indicates the existence of demonstrable differences in the bioavailability of products involving roughly a score of drugs. A partial list of studies demonstrating bioinequivalence of chemically equivalent drug products might include the following: tetracycline[2, 3]; chloramphenicol[4]; digoxin[5, 6]; phenylbutazone[7, 8]; and oxytetracycline[9, 10]. Not only has bioinequivalence been shown to exist in products of different manufacturers but there also have been substantial variations in the bioavailability of different batches from the same company[6].

It is difficult to determine whether differences such as those cited are the exception or the rule, since positive results (in this case a demonstrable difference) are far more likely to be published than negative findings. Furthermore, in some studies in which several chemically equivalent products have been tested, some have been found to have the same bioavailability while others have not.

Bioequivalence testing usually arises when a patent on an innovator's drug expires. Other manufacturers may then wish to market the same formulation of the drug. Formulations that are bioequivalent with that of the innovator and bearing the generic name of the drug are called generic products. The objective of bioequivalence testing is to assure therapeutic equivalence of generic products to innovator products. Bioequivalence testing is also performed during the course of development of new drugs, when a formulation is changed or when the site or method of manufacture is altered [11].

Laws mandate the new drug products be safe and effective. If a new product of a drug has the same molar dose and is of similar formulation to one already shown to be safe and effective, such laws allow marketing of the new product if it shows bioequivalence *i.e.*, similar efficacy and safety.

Bioequivalence determinations usually carried out by administering reference and test dosage forms to a group of healthy human subjects, followed by collection and assay of blood (plasma or serum) samples. It is based on the assumption that two dosage forms that exhibit superimposable plasma concentration time profiles in a group of subjects should result in identical therapeutic activity in patients. The key parameters to note from Plasma concentration time profile are the peak concentration (C_{max}), time of occurrence of peak concentration (T_{max}) and the total area under the plasma concentration time curve (AUC).

Time of peak concentration (T_{max}) is the time required to achieve the peak plasma concentration after single dose administration of the drug. The value of T_{max} provides a means to assess the rate of absorption of the drug. The T_{max} is independent of the amount of drug absorbed but is inversely related to the absorption rate. Thus, the faster the absorption of a drug, the shorter will be the T_{max}. The value of T_{max} is also influenced by the rate of elimination of the drug from the body. However, if one assumes elimination rate does not change during the period when two or more jdosage jforms are being tested in a given subject, then observed differences in T_{max} will reflect absorption rate differences among the test products.

Peak concentration (C_{max}) represents the highest concentration attained by the drug in the plasma. At C_{max}, the rate of drug elimination becomes equal to rate of drug absorption. The interpretation of C_{max} is somewhat more complecated because it is a function of both the rate of absorption and the extent of absorption, as well as the elimination rate. Thus, as the amount of drug absorbed increases and/or the rate of absorption increases, the C_{max} also increases, assuming no change in elimination rate.

Total area under the curve (AUC) is related to the extent of drug absorption. Thus, it is directly proportional to the fraction of the administered dose that reaches the systemic circulation. However, changes in AUC may not necessarily reflect changes in the total amount of drug absorbed, but the modifications in the kinetics of distribution, metabolism and excretion of the drug as well. The calculation of AUC is commonly accomplished using the linear trapezoidal rule.

DESIGN AND CONDUCT OF BIOEQUIVALENCE STUDY

In the following sections, requirements for the design and conduct of bioequivalence studies are formulated. The design should be based on a reasonable knowledge of the pharmacodynamics and/or the pharmacokinetics of the active substance in question. In general, single dose studies will suffice, but there are situations in which steady-state studies may be required:

(a) if problems of sensitivity preclude sufficiently precise plasma concentration measurement after single dose;

(b) if the intra-individual variability in the plasma concentrations or disposition rate is inherently large;

(c) in the case of dose- or time-dependent pharmacokinetics;

(d) in the case of extended release products (in addition to single dose studies).

In such steady-state studies the administration scheme should follow the usual dosage recommendations. It would seem that multiple dosing would be the logical choice for drugs intended for long-term use since this would give a more realistic comparison in view of the way in which the drug is normally administered. Other advantages of conducting a multiple-dose study over a single-dose study include:

1. Multiple-dosing eliminates the long washout periods required between single-dose administrations. The switch-over from one formulation to the other can take place in steady state.

2. Single-dose studies may pose problems of sufficiently long sampling periods in order to get reliable estimates of terminal half-life, which is needed for correct calculation of the total AUC.

3. Multiple-dose studies yield higher concentrations of drug in the blood, making accurate measurement easier. In addition, since drug concentrations need to be measured only over a single dosing interval at steady state, the need to measure lower concentrations during a disposition phase is avoided.

4. Multiple-dosing studies can be conducted in patients, rather than healthy volunteers, allowing the use of higher doses.

5. Usually, smaller intersubject variability is observed in steady-state studies, which may permit the use of fewer subjects.

6. Nonlinear pharmacokinetic, if present, can be more readily detected at steady-state following multiple-dosing.

On the other hand, multiple-dose bioequivalence studies are undesirable in some respects. Healthy subjects should not be dosed with any drug for an extended period of time. Multiple-dose studies are also generally more difficult to carry out, especially with regard to ensuring subject compliance with dosing and dietary restrictions. Therefore, most bioequivalence studies are conducted as single-dose studies. Multiple-dose studies should be performed only when a single-dose study is not a reliable indicator of bioavailability.

Design

The design and analysis of clinical trials is fertile soil for statistical applications. The proper design of a bioavailability or bioequivalence study is essential to the collection of meaningful data. For example, both types of studies must include a sufficient number of subjects and require blood or urine samples at appropriately spaced intervals. In a bioequivalence study involving two or more dosage forms, the sequence of product administration must be carefully considered to minimize experimental bias. It is essential to adopt a double-blind technique where both the observer and patient (or subject) are unaware of the treatment being given during the course of study. Manufacturing alternative treatment dosage forms to be as alike as possible in terms of shape, size, color, odor, and taste accomplish the double-blind method. Randomization is an integral and essential part of the implementation and design of bioequivalence studies. Randomization will help to reduce potential bias in clinical experiments.

There are two types of study designs adaptable for bioequivalence studies; they are Parallel design and Crossover design. In a parallel design, two or more drug products are studied, drug products being randomly assigned to different patients. Each patient is assigned a single drug.

In a crossover design, each subject receives each of the drug products under investigation on different occasions. Perhaps the greatest appeal of the crossover design is that patient acts as his or her own control. In such a design, differences among dosage forms, subjects, and sequences of administration can be readily estimated. However, caution should be used when considering this design in studies where carryover effects or other interactions are anticipated. Under these circumstances, a parallel design may be more appropriate.

The crossover or (changeover) design is a very popular, and often desirable, design in clinical experiments like bioequivalence studies. Using this method, both the test and the reference products are compared in each subject, so that inter-subject variables, such as age, weight, differences in metabolism, etc., are minimized. Each subject thus acts as his own control. Also, with this design, subjects daily variations are distributed.

In crossover designs, the test and reference dosage forms, are compared, with each patient or subject taking each dosage form in turn. The dosage forms are taken in two occasions. The administration of each dosage form is followed by a sufficiently long period of time to ensure complete elimination of the drug (washout period) before the next administration. The order of administration is randomized; that is, either B follows A or A follows B, where A & B are the two dosage forms.

A ————————————→ B   or   B ————————————→ A
First week   First week   First week   First week

Since each patient takes each product, the comparison of the products is based on within-patient variation. Thus crossover experiments usually result in greater precision than the parallel-groups design, where different patients comprise the two groups. Given an equal number of observations, the crossover design is more powerful than a parallel design in detecting product differences. Also, the crossover is usually more economical: one-half the number of subjects has to be recruited to obtain the same number of observations in a parallel design. There are also some problems associated with crossover designs. A crossover study may take longer to complete than a parallel study because of the extra testing period. Perhaps the most serious problem with the use of crossover design is differential carryover or residual effect.

The features of the two-period crossover design follow:

1. N subjects recruited for the study are separated into two groups or two treatment sequences. N_1 subjects take the drug products in the order AB and N_2 in the order BA, where $N_1 + N_2 = N$. For example, 24 (N) subjects are recruited and 12 (N_1) take the generic followed by brand product, and 12 (N_2) take the brand followed by the generic.

2. After administration of the product in the first period, blood levels of the drug are determined at suitable intervals.

3. A wash-out period follows, which is of sufficient duration to ensure the "total" elimination of the drug given during the first period. An interval of atleast nine drug half-lives should be sufficient to ensure virtually total elimination of the drug. Often a minimum of 7 half-lives is recommended.

4. The alternative product is administered in the second period and blood levels determined as during period 1.

Crossover designs are planned so that each treatment is given an equal number of times in each period. This is most efficient and yields unbiased estimates of dosage form differences if a period effect is present.

Subjects

A single-dose bioequivalency studies is generally performed in normal, healthy, adult volunteers. If feasible, taking into account reproduction toxicology, they should belong to both sexes and be between 18 and 55 years old. In the case of genetic polymorphism in clearance it is wise to take this into consideration in selecting subjects. In some cases the toxic character of the active substance studied may be such that only patients—under suitable precautions and supervision—can be studied. In that case the applicant will have to justify his alternative. The subject population should be selected carefully, so that product formulations , and not intersubject variations, will be the only significant determinants of bioequivalence. A minimum of 12 subjects is recommended, although 18 to 24 subjects are used to increase the data base for statistical analysis. The test and reference products are usually administered to the subjects in the fasting state (overnight fast for at least 10 hours, plus 2 to 4 hours after administration of the dose), unless some other approach is more appropriate for valid scientific reasons. Time and preferably composition of meals taken after the treatment should be standardised. Because fluid intake may profoundly influence gastric passage, it should be strictly standardised and specified. The subjects should not take other medicines for one week prior to the study and during the study. They should preferably abstain from food and drinks which may interact with circulatory, gastro-intestinal, liver or renal function (*e.g.* alcoholic or xanthine-containing beverages). Preferably they should be non-smokers. If smokers are included they should be identified as such. In some cases (*e.g.* study of high clearance substances) even posture or physical activity may have to be standardised.

Reference and Test Product

All investigative products must have been prepared in accordance with GMP-rules. Batch control results of the test product should be reported. Generic products are normally compared with the corresponding form of a well established "Innovator" medicinal product (reference product). The choice of reference product should be justified by the applicant.

The test product will mostly originate from a test batch. After scale-up samples of the product from the production batches should be compared with those of the test batch, and they should show the same dissolution rate "*in vitro*" in a discriminatory test. The study sponsor will have to retain a sufficient number of product samples for the accepted shelf life plus one year to allow repetition of "*in vitro*" and "*in vivo*" studies at the request of the authority.

ANALYTICAL METHODS

The conduct of bioavailability studies in man requires that a drug product be administered to a group of individuals and that the time-course of the concentration of the drug in the blood be evaluated either directly or indirectly. It is necessary, therefore, that there be available[1] analytical methods for determining the concentration of the active ingredient in body fluids;[2] standardized procedures for administering the drug product and obtaining appropriate blood and/or urine samples; and[3] adequate methods for statistical analysis and interpretation of the results.

The bioanalytical methods used to determine the active principle and/or its biotransformation products in plasma, serum, blood or urine or any other suitable matrix should meet requirements of specificity, accuracy, sensitivity and precision. Knowledge of the stability of the active substance and/or its biotransformation product in the sample material is a prerequisite for obtaining reliable results.

Generally evaluation of bioequivalence will be based upon the measured concentrations of the active substance. If this is impossible a major biotransformation product should be used. The measurement of concentrations of biotransformation product is essential if the substance studied is a prodrug. If urinary excretion (rate) is measured the product determined should represent a major fraction of the dose, and the excretion rate should be considered to parallel plasma concentrations of the active substance.

It may be necessary to measure, in a small volume of biological fluids, an amount of the intact drug that is only one millionth to one billionth of the dose administered. Fortunately, such recent advances as gas-liquid chromatography, high pressure liquid chromatography, fluorescence techniques, mass spectrometry, radioimmuno assays, and microbiological assays have greatly increased our capability of measuring such minute amounts of drugs. The methods used must have not only adequate sensitivity and accuracy, but also the selectivity that will make it possible to quantify the drug in the presence of its metabolites or of endogenous compounds that may interfere with the determination of the compound in biological fluids.

In instances in which no sufficiently sensitive chemical method is available to detect the active ingredient, radioactively labeled molecules may be utilized. It must be verified, however, that the measured radioactivity is contained in the intact compound that has been separated from its metabolites. One must also be assured that the dosage form containing the radioactive drug to be administered possesses, insofar as possible, physical and chemical properties identical to those of the usual (unlabeled) dosage form.

Some of these methods are cumbersome and rather time-consuming, but they are capable of providing relatively accurate measurements at the required levels. Unfortunately, some of the early pharmacokinetic studies were based on methods subject to ambiguities. Continuing efforts, therefore, are still required to simplify and improve the existing methods and to develop new ones.

Characteristics to be Investigated

In order for different formulations of the same drug substance to be considered bioequivalent, they must be equivalent with respect to the rate and extent of drug absorption. Thus, the two predominant issues involved in the assessment of bioequivalence are: the pharmacokinetic parameters that best characterize the rate and extent of absorption and, the most appropriate method of statistical analysis of the data.

With regard to the choice of the appropriate pharmacokinetic characteristics, it is more appropriate that the comparisons of the formulations should be made with respect to only those parameter(s) of the blood level profile that possess some meaningful relation to the therapeutic effect of the drug. Since the AUC is directly proportional to the amount of drug absorbed, this pharmacokinetic parameter is most commonly used to charaterize the extent of absorption, both in single-and multiple-dose studies.

The choice of an appropriate pharmacokinetic characteristic for the rate of absorption is still being discussed with considerable controversy. Although a broad array of methods exists for calculating absorption rates, the most commonly used parameters are peak concentration (C_{max}) and time to peak concentration (t_{max}). Although these parameters have been observed to have significant variances and may be difficult to determine accurately, they remain the parameters generally requested as rate characteristic by most regulatory authorities for immediate-release products.

If pharmacodynamic effects are used as characteristics the measurements should provide a sufficiently detailed time course and the initial values should be the same. Specificity, precision and reproducibility of the measurements should be sufficient. The non-linear character of the dose/response relationship should be taken into account.

General Approach for Single-dose Bioequivalence Study

The following general approaches are recommended for *in vivo* pharmacokinetic Bioequivalence studies,

Study Conduct

○ The test or reference products should be administered with about 8 ounces (240 ml) of water to an appropriate number of subjects under fasting conditions, unless the study is a food-effect BA/BE study.

O Generally, the highest marketed strength should be administered as a single unit. If necessary for analytical reasons, multiple units of the highest strength can be administered, providing the total single-dose remains within the labeled dose range.

O An adequate washout period (*e.g.*, more than 5 half lives of the moieties to be measured) should separate each treatment.

O The lot numbers of both test and reference listed products and expiration date for the reference product should be stated. The drug content of the test product should not differ from that of the reference listed product by more than 5 percent. The sponsor should include a statement of the composition of the test product and, if possible, a side-by-side comparison of the compositions of test and reference listed products. The samples of the test and reference listed product must be retained for 5 years.

O Prior to and during each study phase, subjects should[1] be allowed water as desired except for one hour before and after drug administration;[2] be provided standard meals no less than 4 hours after drug administration;[3] abstain from alcohol for 24 hours prior to each study period and until after the last sample from each period is collected.

Sample collection and sampling times:

O Under Normal circumstances, blood, rather than urine or tissue, should be used. In most cases, drug, or metabolites are measured in serum or plasma. However, in certain cases whole blood may be more appropriate for analysis. Blood samples should be drawn at appropriate times to describe the absorption, distribution, and elimination phases of the drug. For most drugs, 12 to 18 samples, including a predose sample, should be collected per subject per dose. This sampling should continue for at least three or more terminal half lives of the drug. The exact timing for sample collection depends on the nature of the drug and the input from the administered dosage form. The sample collection should be spaced in such a way that the maximum concentration of the drug in the blood (C_{max}) and terminal elimination rate constant (Kel) can be estimated accurately. At least three to four samples should be obtained during the terminal log_linear phase to obtain an accurate estimate of Kel from linear regression. The actual clock time when samples are drawn as well as the elapsed time related to drug administration should be recorded.

The following pharmacokinetic information is recommended for submission:

- O C_{max} (Maximum Plasma Concentration)
- O t_{max} (Time to Maximum Plasma Concentration)
- O $AUC_{(0-t)}$ (Area under plasma concentration time curve 0 to t hours)
- O $AUC_{(0-a)}$ (Area under plasma concentration time curve 0 to α)
- O $t_{1/2}$ (elimination half life)
- O K_{el} (elimination rate constant)

STATISTICAL METHODOLOGY FOR BIOAVAILABILITY STUDIES

After a bioequivalence study is conducted and the appropriate parameters are determined, the pharmacokinetic data must be examined according to a set of predetermined criteria to confirm or refute the bioequivalency of the test and reference formulations. That is, one must determine whether the test and reference products differ within a predefined level of statistical significance. Since the statistical outcome of a bioequivalence study is the primary basis of the decision for or against therapeutic equivalence of two products, it is critically important that the experimental data be analyzed by an appropriate statistical test.

The statistical methods to be used in bioavailability studies should be chosen with careful attention being given to the effect of the variations among individuals and among batches of nominally identical manufactured drug products. The planning, analysis and interpretation of these experiments are not routine problems but, rather, require considerable care, consonant with the purpose for which the data are to be used.

INDIVIDUAL VARIABILITY AND BIOEQUIVALENCE

When drug products are administered to individuals, the investigator inevitably finds differences in one or more of the variables measured. These differences are due partly to factors related to dosage form and partly to biological factors unique to each individual, since each person has his own characteristics for absorption, metabolism and excretion of each drug. Through appropriate use of statistical procedures, it is possible to identify the variations that result from differences among individuals and thus to isolate those that result from differences in the bioavailability of the drug products.

SAMPLE-SIZE CONSIDERATIONS

One of the most important and difficult problems in planning bioavailability investigations is the selection of the appropriate sample size. If conventional statistical tests of significance are used to analyze the data, then it is possible that studies involving small numbers of observations (subjects) may fail to yield differences that are statistically significant even if the drug products being compared are, in fact, different. Alternatively, if large numbers of observations are used, then one may find statistically significant differences between drug products, even if the real differences are small and of no pharmaceutical or therapeutic significance. Therefore, in planning bioavailability investigations, one must determine the difference in mean values of the parameters of bioavialability that it is practically (pharmaceutically or therapeutically) important to detect. The choice of sample size requires that the probability of failing to detect important differences be small, when such differences exist.

METHODS OF DATA ANALYSIS

The experimental results of bioequivalency studies can be analyzed statistically in many different ways. The statistical methods of analysis depend on[1] the statistical model of the concentration-time curve,[2] the statistical model of the various sources of variation (for example, person-to-person variations, or nonindependent measurements), and[3] the experimental plan that specified how the measurements were to be made. Perhaps the simplest way to use concentration-time curves for comparing two drug products is not to compare the entire curves but to compare characteristics of the curves that are deemed important with regard to the drug product under study-for example, area under the curves, peak heights, or rates of absorption. If only a single characteristic is involved, an appropriate method of analysis is the method of paired comparisons, in which each individual generates a paired difference. There are also adequate statistical procedures for the comparison of two or more sets of variables, and these, can be used when more than two drug products are studied.

Statistical Analysis

In the early 1970s, bioequivalence was usually determined only on the basis of mean data. Mean AUC and C_{max} values for the generic product had to be within ±20% of those of the reference product. Although the 20% value was somewhat arbitrary, it was felt that for most drugs, a 20% change in the dose would not result in significant differences in the clinical response to drugs. A relatively common misconception is that current regulatory standards still allow this difference of 20% in the means of the pharmacokinetic variables (C_{max} and AUC) of the test and reference formulations. The FDA's statistical criteria for approval of generic drugs now requires the application of confidence limits to the mean data, using an analysis known as the two one-sided tests procedure.

A test formulation was considered to be bioequivalent to a reference formulation if

$$0.8 < \frac{AUC_{test}}{AUC_{ref}} < 1.2$$

and

$$0.8 < \frac{C_{max\ test}}{C_{max\ ref}} < 1.2$$

By this procedure, if test and reference products were not bioequivalent (*i.e.* means differed by more than 20%), there was a 5% chance of concluding that they are bioequivalent. The current FDA guidelines are that two formulations whose rate and extent of absorption differ by 20%/+25% or less are generally considered bioequivalent. In order to verify that the 20%/+25% rule is satisfied, the two one-sided statistical tests are carried out: one test verifies that the bioavailability of the test product is not too low and the other to show that it is not too high. The current practice is to carry out the two one-sided tests at the 0.05 level of significance. Computationally, the two one-sided tests are carried out by computing a 90% confidence interval. For approval, a generic manufacturer must show that the 90% confidence interval for the ratio of the mean response (usually AUC and C_{max}) of its product to that of the reference is within the limits of 0.8 to 1.25.

Since these tests are carried out at the 0.05 level of significance, there is no more than a 5% chance that they will be approved as equivalent if they differ by as much or more than is allowed by the equivalence criteria (20%/+25%).

Since this test requires that the 90% confidence interval of the difference between the means be within a range of 20%/+25%, it is more stringent than simply requiring the comparison of the test and reference products' AUC and C_{max} to be within the 80 to 125% range. If the mean response of the generic product in the study population is near 20% below or 25% above the innovator mean, one or both of the confidence limits will fall outside the acceptable range and the product will fail the bioequivalence test. Thus, the confidence interval requirement ensures that the difference in mean values for AUC and C_{max} will actually be less than 20%/ +25%. It should be pointed out that the standards vary among drugs and drug classes. For example, antipsychotic agents may fall within a 30% variation and antiarrhythmic agents may be allowed a 25% variation.

Controversies and Concerns in Bioequivalence

The design, performance and evaluation of bioequivalence studies have received a great deal of attention over the past decade from academia, the pharmaceutical industry and regulatory agencies. A number of concerns and questions have been raised about the conduct of bioequivalence studies as well as the guidelines and criteria used to determine bioequivalence.

Most of the concerns of the scientific community centered around adequate standards for evaluation of bioequivalence and correlation between bioequivalence and therapeutic equivalence.

Regulatory attempts to establish specific criteria for judging bioequivalence has generated an exciting and, at times, heated debate mainly because of the evolving nature of the topic and its wide implications.

A main topic of criticism is the statistical design used for the analysis of bioequivalence data. Assessment of bioequivalence was done on the basis of mean data: mean AUC and C_{max} values for the generic product had to be within +20% of those of the innovator product for approval. A statistical test was employed to assess the power of the test to detect a 20% mean difference in treatments. For drugs that could not meet the statistical criteria because of inherent variability, another rule was used, the so-called "75/75" rule: that in at least 75% of the subjects, the test formulation must fall within the range of 75% to 125% of the reference standard to be considered equivalent. Some studies have shown that the rule may accept dissimilar products or reject similar products especially when the study suffers from large inter-, or intra-subject variability.

The second major area of controversy has focused on the criteria used to determine bioequivalence. Implicit in the FDA guidelines is the assumption that a 20%/+25% change in mean serum concentration of drugs can be safely tolerated. However, there is little documentation demonstrating whether 20% variation in bioavailabilities does or does not affect the safety and efficacy of drugs. There are certain critical therapeutic categories (cardiovascular drugs, Anticonvulsants, Bronchodilating agents and Oral anticoagulants) in which minor fluctuations in blood levels may have a substantial impact on therapeutic outcome or toxicity. In view of this, it has been recommended to lower the variability to ±10%, or to set individual limits based on the pharmacological properties of the drug being studied.

The third criticism of bioequivalence testing is that it is almost always done in a panel of young, healthy male volunteers rather than in the target population for which the drug is intended. Clearly, the performance of a drug product in a 20-year-old male will not be the same as in an 85-year-old woman. Serious concerns have been raised that different results would be observed in elderly patients, in women, in patients with diseases of the gastrointestinal tract, and in patients with diminished renal or hepatic function. However, although factors such as age and disease state might affect the actual observed concentrations of drug, the products being compared should be affected in a similar fashion, and one can still be compared to the other. If two products show an equivalent level in healthy volunteers, their levels should be elevated to the same extent in patients with impaired hepatic function. Thus, they can still be compared to each other. Healthy male volunteers are generally used in bioequivalence studies to assure a homogeneous study population and to permit focus on formulation factors that might affect bioavailability. In addition, healthy subjects are more likely to remain stable during the study. The condition of actual patients might change due to the disease resulting in greater variability in the data.

A fourth source of controversy in bioequivalence is the very foundation on which the whole concept of bioequivalence is based: the central assumption is that if two products are shown to be bioequivalent by currently accepted standards, then they are also therapeutically equivalent, and thus interchangeable. A number of critics have challenged this "bioequivalence = therapeutic equivalence" equation, pointing out that this relationship has not been conclusively established for most drugs. These terms are, in fact, not interchangeable; bioequivalence means that two products have basically superimposable blood level curves (within specified limits) while therapeutic equivalence means the products produce similar effects. There may be situations where two products have similar blood concentrations, yet if the drug has a narrow therapeutic range, they may have significantly different therapeutic effects. On the other hand, there may be products, which have widely varying blood level profiles, but exhibit very little difference in their clinical effect. This might be the case for drugs with a wide therapeutic range. In addition, the therapeutic efficacy of some drugs is not necessarily related to their blood levels, e.g., some psychoactive drugs, where the end point of drug effects is psychological and behavioral response.

Williams suggests several ways that the integrity of a bioequivalence study as a prediction of therapeutic equivalence could be assessed. One way involves the performance of specific clinical studies to confirm that products shown to be bioequivalent in healthy subjects would be bioequivalent in the patient population as well. A second way suggested is through post-marketing surveillance of therapeutic response produced by different formulations of the same drug under actual conditions of use. A third method is based on anecdotal reports. Williams points out that none of these methods have been systematically employed to confirm current bioequivalence methodology.

Thus, a number of problems remain in the bioequivalence process which should be addressed. However, a great deal of progress has been made in this area in the last twenty years. The improved design of the studies, the interpretation of the data, the increased scientific rigor of the acceptance criteria, as well as the more rigorous auditing and inspection program have made bioequivalence data an appropriate and valid means of approving generic drug products.

REFERENCES

1. Notari, R. E. (1987). *Biopharmaceutics and Clinical Pharmacokinetics: An Introduction*, 4th edition, Marcel Dekker, New York.
2. MacDonald, H., Pisano, F., Burger, J., Dornbush, A., and Pelcak, E. (1969). Physiological availability of various tetracyclines. *Clinical Medicine*, (Dec) pp. 30-33.
3. Barr, W. H., Gerbracht, L. M., Letchen, K., Plaut, M. and Strahl, N. (1972). Assessment of the biological availability of tetracycline products in man. *Clin. Pharmacol. Ther.*, **13**(1): (Jan./Feb.) 97-108.
4. Glazko, A. J. (1971). Diphenyhydantoin. Panel Discussion on Case Histories in Bioavailability of Drugs, the Proceedings of the Conference on the Bioavailability of Drugs, Washington, United States Pharmacopeial Convention, Inc., pp. 163-177.
5. Wagner, J. G., Wilkinson, P. K., Sedman, A. J., and Stoll, R. G. (1973). Failure of USP tablet disintegration test to predict performance in man. *J. Pharm. Sci.*, **62**(5): (May) 859-860.
6. Lindenbaum, J., *et al.* (1971). Variations in biological availability of digoxin from four preparations. *N. Eng. J. Med.*, **285**: 1344.
7. Van Petten, G. R., Feng, H., Withey, R. J., and Lettau H. F. (1971). The physiological availability of solid dosage forms of phenylbutazone. *J. Clin. Pharmacol.*, **11**: (May/June), 177-196.
8. Choiu, W. L. (1972). Determination of physiological availability of commercial phenylbutazone preparations. *J. Clin. Pharmacol.*, **12**: (July), 296-299.
9. Blair, D. C., Barnes, R. W., Wildner, E. L., and Murray, W. J. (1971). Biological availability of all manufacturing sources supplying the United States market. JAMA, **215**(2): (Jan. 11) 251-254.
10. Brice, G. W. and Hammer, H. F. (1969). Therapeutic non-equivalency of oxytetracycline capsules. *Drug Information Bulletin*, (Jan/June), pp. 112-114.
11. Rowland, M., and Tozer, T. N. (1996). *Clinical Pharmacokinetics Concepts and Applications*, 3rd edition, B.I. Waverly Pvt. Ltd., PA.

9

INTRODUCTION TO BIO-ANALYTICAL METHOD DEVELOPMENT AND VALIDATION FOR BIO-AVAILABILITY AND BIO-EQUIVALENCE STUDIES

T. Nageshwar Rao*

INTRODUCTION

Bio-analytics is the application of analytical technique to determine drug or metabolite concentrations in biological matrix samples mostly in plasma, serum or urine samples related to Bio-availability and Bio-equivalence studies.

It plays a key role throughout the drug development from discovery to drug approval.

The field of bio-analytics covers a wide cross-section of modern analytical techniques and advanced equipments. It is very important to decide whether we require to estimate only analyte(s) or metabolite (s) or both before starting method development.

Before starting the method development a full literature survey has to be completed by using internet or book references, for molecular weight, structure, solubility and stability, type of the instrument and technique required and their availability, type and volume of matrix required.

The useful internet site for literature survey is www.ncbi.nlm.nih.gov/entrez, useful journals (Jrl.) are Jrl. of chromatography B and Jrl. of mass spectroscopy and books like HPLC methods for pharmaceutical analysis by Lunn and schmuff.

Sometimes it is required to collect more amount of matrix or to increase the dose of the formulation, if the analytical method fails to achieve the desired sensitivity. At the same time the literature survey should focus on whether any precautions required during collection of blood like protection from UV light or adding of any stabilizing agent or anti-oxidant or derivatization of the analyte has to be done.

It is also very important to make sure that all the analytical instruments and glasswares like HPLC or LC-MS-MS or GC or GC-MS-MS, pipettes, centrifuge, volumetric flasks, balance, MilliQ water plant, Spectrophotometer

*Group Leader, Clinical Research, 142 IDA Cherlapally, Vimta Labs Ltd., Hyderabad.

etc. which are required to develop a method have to be properly validated and calibrated.

The environmental conditions, water and standards used for method development also have some influence. The environmental conditions like temperature (should be 22°C ± 1°C for LC MS or GC MS and 25°C ± 2°C for others.) and humidity should be around 50 to 75. The water used for bio-analytical purpose should be USP grade except for cleaning. It is important to have a certificate of analysis mentioning the extent of purity, storage condition, manufacturer name and address and date of expiry for all the standards used.

Important instruments used for bio-analytics are

- ○ High Performance Liquid Chromatography (HPLC)
- ○ Liquid Chromatography with Mass Spectroscopy (LC-MS-MS)
- ○ Gas Chromatography (GC)
- ○ Gas Chromatography with Mass Spectroscopy (GC-MS-MS)

Other Supplementary Equipments Required Are

- ○ UV Visible Spectrophotometer
- ○ Electronic Balance
- ○ Freezers
- ○ Refrigerated Centrifuges
- ○ pH meter
- ○ Sample concentrators (Evaporators)
- ○ Vortex mixers
- ○ Sample shakers
- ○ Pipettes
- ○ Vacuum manifolds etc.

FACTORS AFFECTING RETENTION TIME, SELECTIVITY AND SENSITIVITY

- ○ Type of the instrument used
- ○ Selection of HPLC or GC column
- ○ pH of the mobile phase buffer
- ○ Composition of mobile phase
- ○ Column oven temperature
- ○ Sample injection volume
- ○ Extra column volume
- ○ Sample preparation technique

INSTRUMENT USED

S. No.	HPLC	LC-MS-MS	GC-MS-MS
1	This instrument is not much costlier	It is 10 to 20 times costlier than HPLC	It is 4 to 6 times costlier than HPLC
2	It requires more time to develop a method	It requires less time to develop a method	It requires time and also many times dervatization of the analyte
3	Run times are usually 8 to 20 minutes	Run times are usually 1.8 to 2.5 minutes	Run times are usually 12 to 20 minutes
4	Any type of mobile phase buffers can be used	Mobile phase buffers should be volatile	It requires only Helium as a carrier gas
5	Depending upon the nature of the molecule UV Visible, Fluorescence or ECD detectors can be used	This technique is combination of HPLC and Mass detector	This technique is combination of GC and Mass detector
6	Selectivity and sensitivity is very difficult to achieve	Selectivity and sensitivity achievement is easier	Selectivity and sensitivity achievement is easier but requires special precautions
7	It is not possible to develop a method for all kinds of analytes	For all almost all analytes a method can be developed	Only for volatile and thermally stable analytes
8	The dimensions of the columns used for separation usually 4.6 × 150 to 300 mm	The dimensions of the columns used for separation usually 2.1 to 4.6 × 50 to 75 mm	Usually it is 30 meters in length
9	Difficult to develop a method for combination of analytes in a single run	It is easier	It is easier if the analytes are of same nature
10	In this techniques special gases are not required	In this technique gases like nitrogen, zero air and compressed air are required	Only Helium gas is required
11	Usually sample injection volume will be 20 to 100 µL	Here it is less than 40 µL	Here it is less than 5 µL
12	It requires minimum training	It requires a special expertise	It also requires a special expertise
13	On-line sample processing and injection not much useful	On-line sample preparation and injection increases through put	Solid phase micro extraction available for some kind of molecules

SELECTION OF COLUMN

Depending upon the nature of the analytes reverse phase or normal phase columns for HPLC can be selected. It is very important that these columns should be purchased from authorized suppliers only and the column performance should be done as per the manufacturer certificate or as per the SOP of the lab.

Some of the examples for reverse phase columns are C18, C8, and C4 etc. and for normal phase columns are CN, amino, silica etc.

The commonly used dimensions are:

S.No.	Instrument	Length (mm)	Width (mm)	Particle Size (μ)	Plates (per meter)
1	HPLC	150 to 300	4 to 4.6	5 to 10	50,000
2	LC MS MS	50 to 75	2 to 4.6	3	
3	GC	30 meters	0.25	0.25	3000 (capillary)

In maximum cases the retention time and length of column are inversely proportional. It is very important to note that if the length of column is increased better selectivity and resolution are obtained but sensitivity and peak shape may decrease. The decrease in particle size will give the good peak shape but at the same time the life of the column decreases. It is very important to decide type and dimensions of the column to develop a good method.

It is also found that high carbon loaded columns can be used instead of increasing the length of column for complicated analytes. It is always suggested to use guard columns to avoid damage to the main analytical column.

Column care: HPLC columns should always be stored and washed as certified. In case of reverse phase HPLC columns it is suggested that washing with 100% water to remove the buffers which are present in the column (otherwise they may crystallize and lead to clogging of the column) and then with the required organic solvent(s) in reverse conditions to remove the water otherwise it may lead fungal growth in the column. If the column is not in use it should be capped after washing.

Column Regeneration Procedure

For silica columns: Around 50 ml of the following solvents are pumped at a rate of 1 to 2 mL per minute.

○ Tetrahydrofuran

○ Methanol

○ 2 to 4% aqueous acetic acid

○ 2 to 4% aqueous pyridine

○ Tetrahydrofuran

○ Tert. Butyl methyl ether

For Reverse Phase Columns: Around 50 mL of the following solvents are pumped at a rate of 1 to 2 mL per minute.

○ Water + 4 × 100 μL of dimethyl sulphoxide injected

○ Methanol

○ Chloroform

○ Methanol

SELECTION OF BUFFERS FOR HPLC

The molarity and pH of the buffer used plays a major role in better selectivity, sensitivity and for resolution. The pH range required for buffers is 2.5 to 7.5 depending upon the nature of the analyte, in maximum cases in reverse phase HPLC decrease in pH decrease the retention time and increases the peak shape but at the same time it may affect selectivity and resolution.

It is always better to use 1 to 20milli molar buffer. The increase in molarity of the buffer may give good separation but it decrease the peak shape, sensitivity and column life.

The conventional buffers for HPLC are sodium acetate, sodium dihydrogen phosphate, potassium dihydrogen phosphate, ammonium dihydrogen phosphate, tris buffers etc. Some times along with these buffers it is also advised to use ion pairing agents like butane, pentane, heptane sulfonic acids in various proportions to retain the ionizable analytes on reverse phase HPLC columns.

For LC MS the volatile buffers like 0.1% acetic acid, 0.1% formic acid, ammonium acetate or formate.

Better results are obtained by adjusting the pH of the buffer with conjugated acid or base as per the requirement.

After the preparation of the buffers it is ultra sonicated for easy dissolving of the salt and degassing and then the buffer is filtered through 0.2 μ membrane filter. These buffers are always stored in glass containers to avoid fungal growth and are used within 48 hours.

COMPOSITION OF THE MOBILE PHASE

The composition of the mobile phase is mainly depends on the type of matrix, instrument, column used and number of the analytes to be estimated.

Generally in case of LC MS the proportion of the organic solvent is very high compared to HPLC technique. In many cases the increase in proportion of the organic solvent increases the peak shape and sensitivity but at the same time it may decrease the selectivity and resolution.

In case of some analytes the change in small proportions of composition also affects the retention time and selectivity to a great extent.

Some of the solvents suggested for reverse phase HPLC are acetonitrile and methanol or both in various proportions and for normal phase propanol, water etc.

The below flow chart shows the direction of decreasing polarity and increasing elution power of the solvents

Methanol - Acetonitrile- Ethanol - Isopropanol - Dimethyl formamide - Dioxane

The mobile phase also should be stored in glass containers ant it should be used within 24 hours or upto 48 hours after filtration only.

Some times in HPLC the mobile phase may be used in gradient composition for better separation and resolution and to decrease the total run time.

During method development it is advised not to mix the buffer and solvent together in large proportions unless until binary or quaternary HPLC pumps are available to avoid wastage of the solvent.

It is also suggested to use allegation method for method development. Example if you have prepared 50% of solvent and 50% of buffer and if you want to increase the solvent ratio to 65% simply follow the method as given below:

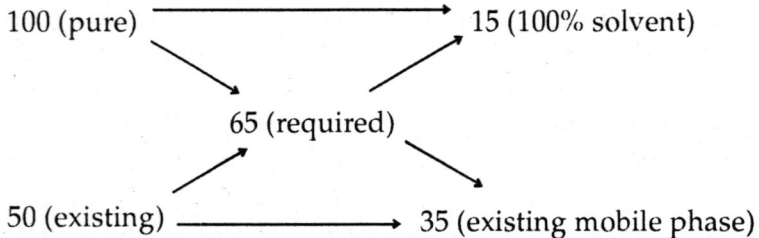

The above method is only for qualitative purpose and during finalization of method fresh mobile phase has to be prepared as required.

COLUMN OVEN TEMPERATURE

When optimized column oven temperature used, it will give good reproducibility in retention time of analyte. Some analytes require higher temperature for elution above ambient temperature. The increase in temperature may decrease the retention time of the analyte and increases the peak shape but at the same it may affect on the selectivity and resolution.

Increasing the temperature, decreases the mobile phase viscosity and allowing higher flow rates and it also increases the diffusivity there by decreasing the resistance to mobile phase mass transfer (analyte molecules diffuse through the mobile phase faster at higher temperatures)

Some of the disadvantages by increasing the temperature:

○ Solvent or sample components are likely to decompose

○ The vapour pressure of the solvent rises, thus increases the risk of bubbles in the detector, which inturn produce an uneven baseline and ghost peaks

SAMPLE INJECTION VOLUME

Sample injection volume does not affect the retention time of the analyte but it has affect on selectivity, sensitivity, peak shape and column life. The increase in sample injection volume may increase the sensitivity but it may decrease the peak shape and column life. It is suggested to decrease the the sample injection volume unless until it is required. Some times if you increase the injection volume the impurities may merge in the analyte peak.

EXTRA COLUMN VOLUME

All volumes within an HPLC instrument which affects the separation are termed extra column volumes. Volumes of the system which are located before the injector or behind the detector are not extra column volumes. Extra column volumes should be kept as low as possible because they may affect the separation and peak shape. They are one cause of band broadening and of tailing. The tubing length and inner diameter should be as low as possible (exa.: suggested inner diameter of the tubing is 0.17 to 0.25 mm) and fittings must be mounted properly.

SAMPLE PREPARATION

Some of the most useful techniques in bio-analytical method development are given below.

1. Precipitation
2. Liquid liquid extraction
3. Solid phase extraction
4. Miscellaneous

    (i) Solid phase micro extraction
    (ii) Derivatization
    (iii) Filtration

1. Precipitation

This technique mainly depends on precipitation of matrix proteins. The acids like trichloro acetic acid and perchloric acid or solvents like methanol and acetonitrile are used in various proportions to precipitate the proteins. This method is not advisable for LC-MS / GC-MS methods.

Procedure

In case of acids: Take 0.5 to 1.0 mL of plasma/serum/ urine and add 100 to 200 µL of 10 to 20% perchloric acid or trichloroacetic acid or some times decreasing the volume and increasing the percentage of acid is also recommended

In case of solvents: Take 0.5 to 1.0 mL plasma and add 0.5 to 2.0 mL of solvent methanol or acetonitrile.

After adding the acid or solvent vortex the vial for complete precipitation of proteins then centrifuge and inject the supernatant.

It is recommended to filter the sample whenever this technique is used to avoid clogging of the column.

Advantages

○ It is an easy and rapid sample processing technique

○ The cost of this sample processing technique is very less

○ The solvents and acids required for this technique easily available

○ This method is more reproducible

○ This method is more useful when the analytes are not extractable (like sartan's)

Disadvantages

○ Chance of incomplete precipitation of proteins

○ It decreases the life of the HPLC column

○ It decreases the sensitivity (minimum detection level) of a method by dilution affect

○ Some times selectivity may not be obtained

2. Liquid- Liquid Extraction

This technique is based on separation of analytes from interferences by partitioning the analyte in between two immiscible liquids or phases. Here one phase is matrix and another is organic solvent or mixture of solvents.

This liquid, liquid extraction can be achieved by manual shaking or by using commercially available shakers. The analytes extracted into the organic phase are easily recovered by evaporation of the organic solvent under steam of nitrogen or air at low temperature (around 40° to 50°C)

Then the residue is reconstituted in mobile phase (usually 0.2 to 1.0 mL) and injected.

Sometimes analytes require back extraction from organic solvent into some diluted acids like 1 to 2 N hydrochloric acid or sulphuric acid. Then the aqueous layer is separated from the organic solvent and injected.

The solvents used for this extraction are diethyl ether, ethyl acetate, hexane, hexane in isoamyl alcohol, teriatiary butyl methyl ether or some times mixture of these solvents.

The use of diethyl ether as 100% organic solvent is generally avoided for this extraction because the chance of pressure generation in the vial is very high.

Procedure

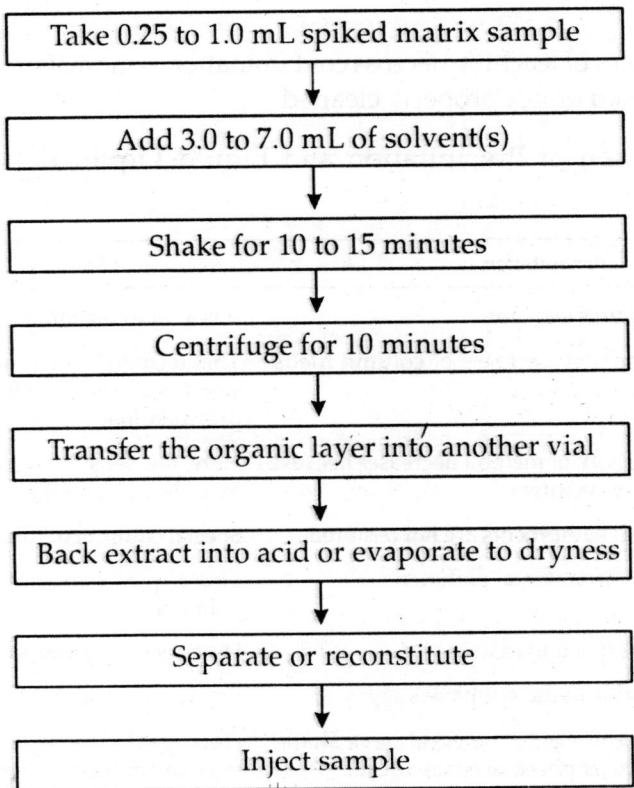

Take 0.25 to 1.0 mL spiked matrix sample
↓
Add 3.0 to 7.0 mL of solvent(s)
↓
Shake for 10 to 15 minutes
↓
Centrifuge for 10 minutes
↓
Transfer the organic layer into another vial
↓
Back extract into acid or evaporate to dryness
↓
Separate or reconstitute
↓
Inject sample

In some cases liquid, liquid extraction after precipitation of proteins is also gives good results. (Procedure: first precipitate the proteins as mentioned in precipitation technique and separate the supernatant and extract as above).

Advantages

○ This method is more selective and sensitive

○ Acceptable percentage recovery achievable

○ This technique is also not too costly

Disadvantages

○ Time consuming process

○ Chance of errors are more and precautions are required

○ Chances of environmental pollution is more

○ It requires special equipments like shakers, evaporators, glassware etc.

○ Chances of leaching or cross contamination is more if proper glassware not used or not properly cleaned

Comparison of Precipitation and Liquid Liquid Extraction (LLE) techniques:

S.No.	Precipitation	LLE
1	It requires less time	It is a time consuming process
2	Chances of decrease of column life is high	This technique may not affect the life of column much, when compared to precipitation.
3	Sensitivity of method decreases because of dilution affect	Here the sensitivity can be increased by concentrating the sample
4	Special equipments are not required	Special equipments are required
5	No environmental pollution	There is a chance of environmental pollution
6	It is simple and easier	Here special precautions are required
7	Filtration of the sample is suggested	Filtration of the sample not required
8	It may not give the good peak shape because of phase reversal affect	Here peak shape is good, because maximum cases the analyte is in mobile phase only

3. Solid Phase Extraction

This technique is covered in separate chapter.

4. Miscellaneous Extraction Techniques

Solid phase micro extraction: This technique is used mainly for GC MS and it is time and temperature dependent, Where the analyte should be thermally stable and volatile. The analyte is adsorbed at particular temperature (which should be less than the boiling point of the solvent in which it is dissolved) Then the pure analytes are desorbed into the port at high temperature in less time. Using this technique we can avoid injecting impurities and we can save the life of column.

Filtration: This technique is mainly useful for urine sample analysis by filtering the sample through suitable filter without extraction.

Derivatization: This technique is useful when analyte is not stable or when the analyte is not having the Ultra violet or fluorescence absorbing properties. It also requires liquid liquid or solid phase extraction before injecting the sample.

METHOD VALIDATION

After developing a method it is advisable that a trial batch containing a calibration curve and quality control checks has to be done before starting a complete method validation.

Bio-analytical method validation includes all of the procedures that demonstrate that a particular method used for quantitative measurement of analytes in a given matrix, such as blood, plasma, serum, or urine, is reliable and reproducible for intended use. The fundamental parameters for this validation include (1) selectivity, (2) sensitivity (3) ruggedness and robustness (4) precision (repeatability), (5) accuracy, (6) recovery (7) linearity (8) stability [In-injector (or) post processing, bench top, freeze-thaw, stock solution short term and long term, matrix samples long term and dilution integrity]

Conduct Full Validation in Case of

- ○ development and implementing a bio-analytical method for the first time
- ○ new drug entity
- ○ validation of revised assay if metabolites are added to an existing assay for quantitation.

Conduct Partial Validation in Case of

○ Bio-analytical method transfers between laboratories

○ Changes in instruments

○ Change in columns

○ Change in matrix within species (e.g. human plasma to human urine)

○ Change in mobile phase ratio etc.

Batch Organization

1 a reference standard solution: containing analyte and ISTD as a mixture or in separate solutions

2 matrix blank

3 matrix blank+ISTD

4 spiked calibration standards (CCs) over the operating range from CC1 to CC7 or CC8

5 QC samples: LLOQ, LQC, MQC & HQC

9 CC's and QC's shall be prepared from different stock solution or same stock with another analyst.

  (*i*) QC of the lower quantitation limit (LLOQ): the same concentration as
CC1

  (*ii*) Low quality control concentration (LQC)-less than or equal 2-3 × CC1

  (*iii*) Medium quality control concentration (MQC)-approximately the mean of LQC and HQC (or) 50% of the largest concentration of the calibration curve (CC7 or CC8)

  (*iv*) High quality control concentration (HQC)-75-90% of the largest concentration of the calibration curve (CC7 or CC8).

The following criteria shall be met for quality control concentrations to be valid

(1) At least three out of six QC samples (50%) at any one concentration level should be within 15% of their respective nominal value.

(2) At least four of every six QC samples (67%) should be within 15% of their respective nominal value. Two of the six QC samples (33%) may be out side the 15% of their respective nominal value. In certain situations wider acceptance criteria may be allowed.

Selectivity

○ Analyze samples from the biological matrix (blood, serum, plasma, urine, or other) obtained from six subjects (Preference: four being normal samples, one lipaemic and one hemolytic, under controlled time conditions, food ingestion and other important factors for the study).

○ Any sample of the blank representing significant interference in the period of time of retention of the analyte, metabolite or internal standard, must be rejected. If more than one of the analyzed samples present such interference, new samples of other six subjects must be tested. If more than one of the samples of the group present significant interference in the period of time of the analyte retention, the method must be altered with the purpose of eliminating it

Limit of Quantification (LLOQ)

LLOQ is the lowest concentration that can be measured with acceptable accuracy and precision.

The analyte response at the LLOQ should be at least 5 times the response compared to blank response. Analyte peak (response) should be identifiable, discrete, and reproducible with a CV% ≤ 20% and accuracy of 80-120%.

Recovery (of analyte and internal standard if applicable)

The recovery measures the efficiency of extraction of analytical method within a variation limit. The recovery in an assay is the detector response obtained from an amount of an analyte added to and recovered from the biological matrix, compared to the detector response obtained for the pure authentic standard. Recovery percentages near to 100% are desirable, nevertheless lower values are accepted, for example, 50 to 60% provided the recovery is precise and accurate.

Perform recovery experiments in quadruplicate for analyte by comparing the analytical results for extracted samples at three concentrations (equivalent to LLOQ, MQC and HQC) with unextracted standards that represent 100% recovery. Similarly 6 sets of one concentration of matrix ISTD concentrations (which is used for precision & accuracy in validation) are compared with 6 sets of aqueous ISTD concentrations (same concentration as used in matrix ISTD). Assess % recovery of analyte and ISTD using appropriate chromatographic conditions. Tabulate peak response and calculate % recovery for each concentration with the formula:

% recovery = (mean response of extracted samples/mean response of unextracted samples) * 100

Acceptance criteria:

○ Accept only methods giving > 50% recovery for method validation.
○ CV% of areas of analyte and ISTD shall be ≤ 20%

Ruggedness and Robustness

Perform ruggedness & robustness for changes in the following parameters using a suitable concentration and establish the acceptance criteria for each parameter.

○ pH of mobile phase buffer
○ column (minimum two columns with same make (or) if possible different lot numbers)
○ analyst variation

Linearity

Concentrations of standards will be chosen based on the expected concentrations of the study. A calibration curve consists a blank sample (matrix sample processed without internal standard), blank with ISTD and 7 or 8 non-zero samples covering the expected range. A linear equation will be determined to produce the best fit for the concentration/response relationship.

Make minimum of six (6) calibration curves using 7 or 8 different concentrations and by keeping CC1 and CC7 or CC8 in duplicate (if required)

Acceptance Criteria

○ Maximum allowed deviation of the CC1 from actual concentration shall be ± 20% and standards other than CC1 from actual concentration shall be ±15%.
○ 'r' and 'r^2' shall be 0.99 and 0.98 respectively.
○ At least five out of seven or six out of eight non-zero standards should meet the above criteria, including the CC1 and the calibration standard at the highest concentration (CC7 or CC8). Any two consecutive points shall not be excluded. Excluding the standards should not change the model used.

Precision and Accuracy

Determine precision and accuracy using a minimum of five determinations per concentration level (excluding blank samples). As a minimum, three concentrations representing the entire range of the standard curve should be studied Both intra and inter day precision and accuracy has to be established.

Acceptance Criteria

	Precision	Accuracy
LLOQ	% CV ≤ 20%	± 20% of actual spiked concentration
Other than LLOQ	% CV ≤ 15%	± 15% of actual spiked concentration

STABILITY
Stock Solution Stability (Short Term and Long Term)
Short Term Stability
Determine the stability of stock solutions of analyte and ISTD at room temperature for at-least 6 hours in comparison to initial (zero time) response by injecting suitable number of samples at two concentration levels for analyte and one concentration for ISTD.

% stability = (mean response after 6.00 Hrs/mean zero time response)*100

Long Term Stability
If the stock solutions are refrigerated for the relevant period, document the same. After completion of the desired storage time, the stability will be tested by comparing the instrument response with that of freshly prepared solutions (no. of injections same as short term).

% stability = (mean response after x.x days* fresh stock concentration/ stored at x.x days stock conc.*mean response of freshly prepared samples)*100.

The stability should be in acceptable limit.

Bench-Top (Short Term Room Temperature) Stability
The stability of analyte (in matrix) on bench (outside the freezer) should be studied to know the stability of samples at room temperature from 4 to 24 hrs (based on the expected duration that samples will be maintained at room temperature in the intended study after thawing) by analyzing suitable number of sets of low and high quality control concentrations.

% stability = (mean of conc. at x.x hours/mean of conc. at 0.0 hour)*100

In-Injector (or) Post-Processing Stability
Determine the stability of processed samples (in matrix) based on the resident time before injection/auto sampler resident time, injecting processed samples

at time intervals like 0.0, 3.0 and 6.0 hours depending on analytical run time by injecting suitable number of low and high quality control concentrations.

% stability = (mean of conc. at x.x hour/mean of conc. at 0.0 hour)*100

Freeze Thaw Stability

Determine analyte stability (in matrix) for three freeze and three thaw cycles. Store the minimum of three sets of each of the low and high concentrations at the intended storage temperature for about 24 hours. Thaw one set of QC's unassisted at room temperature and label them as freeze thaw 3rd cycle samples and store back in freezer for at least another 12 hours, Then after 12 hours take 3rd freeze thaw cycle samples as well as one new set of QCs and label them as 2nd freeze thaw cycle samples and thaw the samples at room temperature after complete thawing of samples keep them back in freezer for at least another 12 hours. Then after 12 hours take 2rd and 3rd freeze thaw samples along with another set and label them as 1st freeze thaw samples and thaw at room temperature. After complete thawing analyze all the sets under a fresh calibration curve and calculate the freeze thaw stability.

% stability = (mean of conc. at xx cycle/mean of conc. at first cycle)*100

Long Term Stability in Matrix Samples

Depending on the time required to complete all clinical periods, number of subjects and samples and analytical run time the stability of the sample should be estimated by using a fresh calibration curve with sufficient number of sets of low and high quality control concentrations at various days *e.g.*: 1, 15, 30 and 60 days (based on time between first sample collection and the last date of sample analysis).

% stability = (mean of conc. at x.x days/mean of conc. of day-1)*100

The Acceptance Criteria for all Above Stability Studies of Analyte in Matrix

The back calculated concentrations should be within 85 % - 115% of actual spiked concentration.

And percentage stability should be within 85% - 115%

NOTE: x.x may be number of days/hours/cycles

Dilution Integrity

Perform dilution integrity test for suitable number of samples by diluting 50:50 and 25:75 with matrix blank of highest spiked concentration (1.5 to 1.8 times the CC7 or CC8 concentration).

Dilution Integrity = (mean conc. obtained/actual conc.)*100

Acceptance Criteria

Precision should be within £ 15% and accuracy within 85 - 115%. of actual spiked concentration

Matrix Affect (in case of LC MS MS)

The affect of matrix on the analyte RT should be studied by spiking and analyzing LLOQ concentration in minimum of six (6) different matrix samples. The back calculated values obtained should be within 80 to 120 percentage of actual spiked concentration.

Partial Volume Verification

This is required when the sample required is insufficient for assay procedure instead of declaring as a insufficient sample. This can be done by processing the sample by taking 50 or 75 percentage of spiked matrix sample and remaining volume is diluted with matrix blank.

NOTE:

1. The specific crisis management plan as to be made in method validation SOP, to deal with the failure to meet acceptance criteria for all above parameters.

2. A complete method development and validation log book or file as to be made along with the all the documents or forms required for validation

DEFINITIONS

Accuracy: The degree of closeness of the determined value to the nominal or known true value under prescribed conditions. This is sometimes termed *trueness*.

Precision: The closeness of individual measures of a analyte when the procedure is applied repeatedly to multiple aliquots of a single homogeneous volume of biological matrix

Analyte: A specific chemical moiety being measured, which can be intact drug, biomolecule or its derivative, metabolite, and/or degradation product in a biologic matrix.

Biological Matrix: A discrete material of biological origin that can be sampled and processed in a reproducible manner. Examples are blood, serum, plasma, urine, feces, saliva, sputum, and various discrete tissues.

Recovery: The extraction efficiency of an analytical process, reported as a percentage of the known amount of an analyte carried through the sample extraction and processing steps of the method.

Selectivity: The ability of the bio-analytical method to measure and differentiate the analytes in the presence of components that may be expected to be present. These could include metabolites, impurities, degradants, or matrix components.

Lower Limit of Quantification (LLOQ): The lowest amount of an analyte in a sample that can be quantitatively determined with suitable precision and accuracy

Upper Limit of Quantification: The highest amount of an analyte in a sample that can be quantitatively determined with precision and accuracy
Quality control sample (QC): A spiked sample used to monitor the performance of a bio-analytical method and to assess the integrity and validity of the results of the unknown samples analyzed in an individual batch

Calibration Curve (CC): The relationship between the experimental response value and the analytical concentration (also called a *Standard curve*).

CC1: The lowest point of the calibration curve and it should not be confused with LLOQ. The value variation between LLOQ and CC1 may be in some decimals only.

Internal Standard (ISTD): test compound (s) (*e.g.* structurally similar analog, stable labeled compound) added to both calibration standards and samples at known and constant concentration to facilitate quantification of the target analyte (s)

Blank: A sample of a biological matrix to which no analytes have been added that is used to assess the selectivity and specificity of the bio-analytical method

Matrix Affect: The direct or indirect alteration or interference in response due to the presence of unintended analytes or other interference substances in the sample

Stability: The chemical stability of an analyte in a given matrix under specific conditions for given time intervals

Full Validation: Establishment of all validation parameters to apply to sample analysis for the bio-analytical method for each analyte.

Partial Validation: Modification of validated bio-analytical methods that do not necessarily call for full revalidation.

REFERENCES

Llyod R. Snyder and Joseph, J. *Kirkland. Practical HPLC Method Development* 2nd edition.
Lunn and Schmuff. *HPLC Methods of Pharmaceutical Analysis* (by Wiley-interscience).

US FDA. *Guidance for Industry—Bioanalytical Method Validation*.

(1992). Analytical method validation: Bioavailability, Bioequivalence and pharmacokinetic studies. *Pharmaceutical Research*, **9**(4).

Miller, Crowther. Analytical Chemistry in GMP Environment (Wiley Inter Science).

Vogel's *Text Book of Quantitative Chemical Analysis*, 6th edition.

United States Pharmacopoeia 26 and NF-21, 2003.

Veronika R. Meyer. *Practical High Performance Liquid Chromatography*, 3rd edition, Wiley Publications.

Dr. Iain McGilveray A report for laboratory process validation- advances in bio-analytical validation.

ASTM methods Volume 14.02 E 898-88, June 1990.

ASTM methods Volume 14.03 E 77 -89, June 1990.

ASTM methods Volume 14.02 E 542 -94, June 1990.

Chatwal and Anand. *Instrumental Methods of Chemical Analysis*.

10

HIGH PERFORMANCE LIQUID CHROMATOGRAPHY, AN UPGRADED TECHNOLOGY FOR THE MONITORING OF THERAPEUTIC DRUGS

Subhabrata Dey*

INTRODUCTION

Food chemists involved with different assays appreciate the fact that they are faced with a wide variety of sample matrices from which they are expected to quantify the analaytes. Sample characteristics such as fat, protein, carbohydrates and mineral content, as well as the expected level of the vitamins of interest, all affect the sample preparation approach which chemist may choose.

Human insulin is the first commercial healthcare product by recombinant DNA Technology. Eli Lilly, the producer of this synthetic insulin often relies on HPLC to conform the structure and to determine the potency of synthetic human insulin[1]. The HPLC techniques developed at Lilly can detect proteins that differ by a single amino acid, and HPLC tests show human insulin (recombinant DNA) is identical to pancreatic human insulin, and a mixture of the two, showed that they were superimposable and identical.

High performance liquid chromatography (HPLC) and its derivative techniques have become the dominant analytical separation tools in the pharmaceutical, chemical and food industries, environmental laboratories and in therapeutic drug monitoring. Just few years ago, it was an enormous struggle to obtain a few micrograms of any interferon in pure form. With the rapid application of new techniques of HPLC many interferons have been purified and produced in relatively large amounts[2]. HPLC is that technology in achieving the first purification of human leukocyte interferon and in providing the initial surprising result that the leukocyte interferons were a family of closely related proteins, not a single species. HPLC has been used to purify other interferons as well. At the Schering Corporation in New Jersey, the work of Drs. Alan Levine and Paul. Reichart demonstrates the advantage of HPLC who successfully isolated, purified, identified and quantified genetically engineered biologically active proteins from fermented

*Incharge, HPLC, Chittaranjan National Cancer Institute 37, S.P. Mukherjee Road, Kolkata-700 026.

broths[3]. From these researches it is evident that HPLC is a major contributor in biotechnology research.

Scientists are trying to develop new methods everyday for both qualitative and quantitative analysis of different products from natural sources and they also are trying to develop new drugs. Using this technique different components like glycerol, acetic acid and ethanol in fruit juices can be effectively separated. The degree of microbial defect, the extent of natural fermentation in fruit juices and the amount of sulfite present in various food and beverages can also be analyzed with the help of HPLC. The analysis of alcohols and organic acids are important as these compounds typically play a role in determining the flavor characteristics of beverages. The presence of alcohols in fruit juices can indicate the product deterioration. The technology is one of the most important tools for the analysis of cholesterol in butter and antioxidant in black and green tea. The technology has its importance in the quantitative analysis of caffeine, aspartame, benzoic acid and sorbic acid (CABS) in soft drinks. HPLC is one of such sophisticated technology by means of which we can even measure the biogenic amines in rat brain tissue, in human blood plasma and also in table olives even in the order of nanogram or picogram level. A method for the simultaneous determinationi of eight biogenic amines (tryptamine, beta phenylethylamine, putrescine, cadaverine, histamine, tyramine, spermidine, and spermine) has been developed[1, 2] to study their occurrence in fermented vegetables in more detail.

THEORY

An HPLC system is composed of several modules each with its own function. A sample is normally introduced into the system via an injector form which a flowing stream of solvent, called mobile phase, forces it, through a narrow (0.009 inch id) bore transport tube to the column. The column is a large (2-8 mm d) tube containing small (5-125 µm) particles known as stationary phase. The sample mixture separates as a result of different components adhering to or diffusing into the packing particles. Thus, as the mobile phase is forced through the chromatographic bed, a sample is separated into various zones of sample components. These zones are often referred to as **bands.** The bands continue to migrate through the bed, eventually pass out of the column by the process of **elution**, and pass through any one or a number of detectors provides input to some recording device, say a strip chart recorder and thus a deflection of the pen on the recorder indicates the elution of one or more chromatographic bands. The recorder tracing from the elution of a single band is called a **peak** and the collections of peaks, which result from an injected sample, comprise the **chromatogram**.

Peaks are usually identified by their retention time, which is time required to elute the corresponding band from the column. For proper identification of peaks, an accurate recording device is needed along with a pumping system that will deliver a precise flow rate throughout the separation. The pump accepts solvent from an outside reservoir and forces it at a constant flow rate through the system. When a sample is injected, it is forced through the column separating into bands that elute, pass through detectors, and results in peaks on a chart recorder. To get proper separation, a number of changes to be made such as solvent flow rate, packing material, column length, solvent composition, detector, column diameter etc.

Although the column is the heart of the HPLC instrument and essential to its success, until now no single book has focused on the theory and practice of column technology. The separation mechanisms of samples depend on some characteristics of the column like base material, particle size and shape, specific surface area and pore size, molecular weight, specific pore volume and particle strength etc.

PACKING MATERIALS

Packing for high performance liquid chromatography (HPLC) can be based on either an inorganic ceramic or an organic polymeric substance. The inorganic ceramics generally used are **sillica** and **alumina** while highly cross linked styrene divinylbenzene based and methacrylate based packing are used for **polymeric base material.** Inorganic packings have a high rigidity and do not swell in any solvent but polymeric packings do not have the rigidity of inorganic packings and are more compressible. Solvents and analytes can penetrate the polymer matrix and cause swelling of the particles and results in low efficiency due to reduced transfer.

Silica is the most popular base material for HPLC packings. In addition to the high physical strength that it shares with other packings, silica provides a surface to which a broad range of ligands can be attached using well established silanization technology. With this surface modification technique, packing for reversed phase, ion exchange, hydrophilic interaction or size exclusion chromatography can be prepared. Silica based packings are compatible with a broad range of solvents from polar to non polar. Their weakness is the limited stability in aqueous alkaline mobile pahses. In general, a pH range of 2 to 8 is recommended for the routine use of silica-based packings. Alumina has the same favourable physical properties as silica with the added compatibility of an extended pH range. Like silica, it is very rigid and does not swell or shrink in any solvents. Unlike silica, bounded phases on alumina are not stable in aqueous mobile phases, however, coated alumina have been produced that show excellent pH stability in aqueous systems.

Polymeric packings are compatible with the typical pressures of HPLC. However, their pressure limit is lower than that of the limit of most inorganic packings. The styrene divinylbenzene matrix is very hydrophobic. It is compatible with all mobile phases, including the entire aqueous pH range. The compatibility with strongly acidic and strongly basic eluents allows through cleaning of the packing with NaOH or strong acids. The methacrylate matrix is intrinsically more hydrophilic than styrene divinylbenzene resin, and it can be made very hydrophilic with appropriate modification of the functional groups. For large molecules like proteins or synthetic polymers, the performance of polymeric packings is comparable to ceramic based packings. Therefore polymeric packings are used extensively in separation of natural and synthetic polymers. As with silica-based packings, a broad range of surface chemistry is available for reversed-phase, ion-exchange, hydrophilic-interaction, hydrophobic-interaction or size-exclusion chromatography.

PARTICLE SHAPE, SURFACE AREA, PORE SIZE AND MOLECULAR WEIGHT

Chromatographic packings are generally available in two particle shapes namely irregular shaped and spherical shaped particles. Irregular shaped particles are widely used in many standard analytical methods. An example of μ Bondapak C_{18} (Waters, USA), which is specified in about 50% of the assays in the US Pharmacopoeia. Minimum size usually available is not less than 5 μm in diameter.

The majority of currently available analytical packings are spherical in shape. They are easier to pack than irregular packings. High performance, good column stability and low backpressure can be achieved. The sizes available are generally from 3 μm to 20 μ., the smaller particle size provides the benefit of shorter analysis time. For reproducibility, spherical packings offer the best choice for analytical applications. The availability of larger particle sizes at reduced cost makes irregular shaped packings attractive for preparative applications.

The specific surface area of packing is determined by the size of the structural elements. This size in turn is closely linked to the pore size of the packing. Therefore there is a fundamental relationship between the specific surface area of packing and the pore size. Packings with a small pore size have a large specific surface area and vice a vise. Surface area is often used as a measure for the retentivity or the capacity of packings. The size of analyte molecules increases with molecular weight. If the size of the molecules is about one third of the pore size or larger, mass transport in the pores is severely hindered and low efficiency and peak broadening results.

Under these circumstances, packings with a larger pore size be used. For all standard analytical problems, packings with pore size between about 6 nm and 13 nm are typically used. The larger pore size packings can also be used for peptide separations. For analytes with a larger molecular weight, for example proteins, packings with a 30 nm pore size are more sutitable. But these packings do not work well with smaller molecules due to the reduced surface area. For analytes with a molecular weight of less then 3,000, the smaller pore size shoudl be used. If the molecular weight is larger than 10,000, packings with a pore size of 30 nm should be used. For analytes with a molecular weight between 3,000 and 10,000, both packings may give satisfactory results.

BONDED PHASE AND MODE OF SEPARATION

Most analytical chromatography is carried out using packings whose sorption properties have been modified by attaching a covalently bonded phase to the surface of silica. Alternatively, coating with a chemically stable absorptive layer can modify the surface of packing. Chemically stable bonds between the packing and the ligands that are responsible for retention are only available for silica and polymeric packings. The surface of the packing can easily be derivatized through silanization. The most commonly used HPLC packing is obtained by derivatization of the surface of silica sorbent with a long chain aliphatic silane. The aliphatic chain is 18 carbons long, and the packing is called C_{18} or ODS (for octadecyl silane). However, several other surface derivatizations of silica are also available which result in packings with widely varying properties. Also polymeric packing with a similar range of surface properties are used in HPLC.

Based on the modes of separation the chromatographic packings are classified into main three categories, namely **Normal Phase Chromatography, Reversed Phase Chromatography and Ion Exchange Chromatography.**

Normal Phase Chromatography

Normal phase chromatography is the classical form of chromatography using polar stationary phases and non polar mobile phases. The solute is retained by the interaction of its polar functional groups on the surface of the packing. Classically, non bounded silica and alumina have been used for this application. But today polar bonded phases can be used with the advantages that the bonded phases equilibrate faster, are less sensitive to minute concentrations of water in the mobile phase, yield different selectivities and cause easy recovery of the sample in preparative separations. Normal phase HPLC is used when the analytes are not water solube, or when a volatile mobile phase is desirable, as in mass spectroscopy and some preparative applications. This type of columns can separate positional isomers. LC-CN, LC-NH$_2$. LC-Diol etc have unique selectivity and can be used for the analysis of sugars, fat-soluble vitamins and steroids respectively.

Reversed–Phase Chromatography

Reversed phase chromatography has become the widest range of applications of any HPLC column type and become the most polar mode chromatography. Consequently, when an unknown mixture is to be analyzed, a reversed phase column usually is tried first. In reversed phase chromatography, the stationary phase is non-polar and the mobile phase is polar. Retention in reversed phase HPLC correlates to the hydrophobicity of the analyte, with the most hydrophobic (least polar) analyte in a sample eluting last. Mobile phases usually are mixtures of polar organic solvents and water, with buffers or salts added to control the degree of ionization of the analyte. The packings in reversed phase columns incorporate silica specially treated to reduce the degree of ion exchange and improve the peak shape for basic compounds. These colmns are widely used in pharmaceutical industries. Reversed phase columns with 300 A particle size are also used for analysis of large molecules, such as proteins and large peptides. Other packings for reversed phase chromatography are graphitized carbon and styrenedivinylbenzene packings. The performance of the reversed phase bounded phases depends also on the activity of the residual silanols. Silanols interact with the polar functional group of the solutes. Therefore, packings exhibit differnet selectivity depending on the activity of the silanols. Also, tailing peaks are often observed for basic compounds on packings with a high level of silanol activity. One way of modifying silanol activity is by endcapping, that is reaction with a silanizing reagent that converts the silanols to trimethylsilyl groups. Fully endcapped bonded phases based on high purity silica are recommended for the chromatography of basic analytes.

Ion–Exchange Chromatography

The separation of solutes by their charge is possible by using phases, which contain fixed ionic charges. In the case of silica based ion exchangers, the ionic species are attached to the surface using standard silanization techniques. In the case of polymer based ion exchangers, the ion exchange groups are distributed through the matrix. There are four categories of ion exchangers: strong and weak cation exchangers and strong and weak anion exchangers. Weak ion exchangers are characterized by the fact that the charge is a function of the pH. Exchangers with carboxylic acids as functional groups are an example of weak cation exchangers. Weak anion exchangers comprise primary, secondary and tertiary amines. The Charge of strong ion exchangers is for the most part independent of pH. Quaternary amines form strong anion exchangers, and sulphonic acids are classified as strong cation exchangers. All these functional groups are available on polymeric packing, primarily for the separation of large biomolecules. All but the weak cation exchangers are available on silica. Also, special ion exchangers are available for ion chromatography.

Ion suppression chromatography is another technique widely used for the analysis of organic acids in eluents at low pH. It is simply a subcategory of reversed phase chromatography. Special polymer phases are available for this application.

Factors Affecting Ion Exchange Retention

Retentation is based on the affinity of different ions for exchanges sites and on other solution, parameters such as pH, ionic strength, temperature and type of counter ion.

pH: To decrease retention, change mobile phase pH to form neutral molecule.

Buffer Concentration: To decrease retention, increase buffer (counterion) concentration

Temperature: To decrease retention, increase temperature.

Examples (APPLICATIONS):

Inorganic Ions

Anions Cl^- ; $SO_4^=$, PO_4^3

Cations Ca^{+2}, Na

Organic Acids

Anions: Carboxylic Acids (R—COO—)

Organic Bases

Cations: Amines (R—NH_3^+)

Proteins and Amino Acids, etc.

Ion–Suppression Chromatography

This technique is widely used for the analysis of organic acids in eluents at low pH. It is simple a subcategory of reversed phase chromatography.

The Nature of Bonded Phases

The nature of a bonded phase depends on Carbon Load, Ligand Density, Type of Bonded Phase and Endcapping.

Carbon Load and Ligand Density

The carbon content of packing is determined by elemental analysis. Often the results are reported directly as the carbon load of packing. Form this value and with the knowledge of the specific surface area of the packing and the molecular weight of the bonded ligand, the ligand density can be calculated. The ligand density is usually expressed in $\mu mol/m^2$. It is also sometimes called the surface coverage. The ligand density is a very important measure of the composition of the surface of the bonded phase, and is one of the important parameters determining the selectivity of packing. Packings with a high ligand density tend to be hydrolytically more stable than packings wit a low ligand density.

Bonded Phase and Endcapping

Bonded phases are produced by the chemical reaction of an organosilane with the silica surface. The target is to achieve a uniform mononuclear layer.

Types of Detectors

Depending on the nature of the samples to be analyzed, different detectors are used of which **Photo Diode Array (PDA) detectors; Dual λ Absorbance Detectors, Scanning Fluoresence Detectors and Electrochemical Detectors** are well known.

The **PDA detector** incorporates a uniquely integrated series of software and optics innovations that enable the system to deliver optimal chromatographic and spectral sensitivity, unparalleled reliability, plus unprecedented ease of use. The innovations help chemists to remain current with evolving compound chemistries and new recombinant techniques required testing closely related compounds. The unique characteristics of this detector are to identify definite compound, to detect and quantitate unprecedented tracer impurity, flexible and reliable instrumentation and mid run optimization.

Dual λ Absorbance detector is of superior performance and versatility for HPLC and can help one to perform analytical, preparative or microbore scale HPLC analysis more efficiently. Its unsurpassed sensitivity allows one to detect the smallest impurities. Its extended linear dynamic range provides simultaneous quantitation of major and minor components is a single run. The innovative, built in cuvette holder makes it easier to qualify than traditional UV/VS detectors.

The main features of this detector are the taper slit flow cell, integrated cuvette holder, lamp optimization soft ware, minimum base line noise and exceptional linearity and advanced programmability.

Scanning Fluorescence detector is a high performance unit that provides a high level of sensitivity for spectrofluoremetric analysis. When certain molecules or atoms are exposed to an energy source such as high intensity light, the molecules or atoms absorb the light energy and enter into an excited state. As a molecule or atom moves from this excited state back to its normal stage, some of the absorbed energy is released in the form of photon. This process is called fluorescence, which is a type of luminescence. The atoms and molecules in different elements and compounds emit different levels of fluorscence when exposed to the same energy levels. The scanning fluorescence detector illuminates a sample with a narrow band of high intensity light from a carefully controlled light source. The detector then measures the low levels of fluorescence emitted form the sample. The emitted light is filtered, amplified and converted to electrical signals that can be recorded and analyzed. The scanning fluorscence detector includes an optical design that maximizes sensitivity, microprocessor control for greater versatility and reliability. There is an emission wavelength sweep function to obtain an emission spectrum and an excitation wavelength sweep function to obtain an excitation spectrum, an automatic second order filter to enhance applications in the visible wavelength range and quartz flow cell, permitting measurement of UV fluorsecence.

Electro Chemical Detector is one of the most recently developed detector and the detection theory consists of electrolysis reaction. It differs from other detection methods in that, the analyte undergoes an electrochemical reaction while being detected. Upon elution from the column, the analyte passes through the electrochemical cell, where it undergoes either an oxidation or a reduction at the working electrode. The controlled potentiostat maintains the potential of the working electrode (relative to a reference electrode) at a value, which causes the analyte to electrolyze. Simultaneously it measures the electrolysis current resulting form the oxidation (or reduction) of the ansalyte. This detector is of low noise and of high sensitivity and flexibility that allows a wide range of chromatographic applications, including catecholamines in plasma, carbohydrates, sulfide, iodide, cyanide and other ions.

Application of Electrochemical Detector[4]

Quantitative analysis of Biogenic amines

Liquid chromatography with electrochemical detection is found to be capable of the determination of catecholamines in blood plasma and also form tissue. The procedures are rapid and inexpensive compared to radio enzymatic assay, HPLC with UV or fluoresecence detection. The method is based on reverse phase ion pair separation techniques which improved the efficiency, sensitivity and versatility of the chromatogram of a number of catecholamines that can be detected within a maximum of 15 minutes using specific mobile phase and specific electric potential.

Serum catecholamine levels more accurately represent the temporal changes that can occur in the sympathetic nervous system. The measurement of circulating catecholamines particularly NE and DA may well provide an important clinical monitor of certain diseases in which dysfunctioing of the sympathetic nervour system is implied. The physiologic responses induced by catecholamines involve changes in hormone secretion and in blood flow distribution.

On the other hand serotonin (5 HT) has already been established to be a substance that plays an important role in nervous transmission not only in the central nervous system but also in the peripheral organs including gastrointestinal tract, heart and lung. It is the most common secretary product of carcinoid tumors where serotonin is synthesized by enzymatic modification. Patients with widely metastatic carcinoid tumors may suffer symptoms of protein malnutrition. Serotonin induces intestinal secretion, inhibits intestinal absorption and stimulates intestinal motility. High serotonin levels are likely the cause of diarrhoea in most cases of carcinoid syndrome. It is therefore concluded that, the proper quantification of the catecholamines including 5 HT suggests and challanges to the search and development of neurotoxicity biological markers which offers the greatest promise for application in human biomonitoring.

Amino Acid Analysis

Amino acid analysis is a fundamental process in any protein research. Knowing the amino acid composition of protein/peptide hydrolysates, physiological fluids, and a myriad of other samples is basic information crucial to further study. The key criteria for any analysis method are accurate and precise identification and quantification of the numerous acid species, high sensitivity detection, and low sample consumption.

Many standard protein chemistry protocols such as protein sequencing and HPLC peptide mapping can now be accomplished with sub picomole sample amounts. Amino acid analysis has been assisted in this derive for higher sensitivity by the use of precolumn derivatization reagernts that yield easily detected fluorescent adducts. The most widely used technique for HPLC amino acid analysis in the Pico Tag method (patent of Waters, USA). Precolumn derivatization relies on the coupling reaction of the well known Edman Degradation, the reaction of phynyl isothiocyanate carbamyl (PTC) derivatives. The method is applicable to any sample including protein hydrolysates, phyiological fluids, feeds, foods and pharmaceutical preparations.

Pico Tag Derivatization Reaction

$$\bigcirc\!\!-\!N=C=S+NH_2-\overset{\overset{\displaystyle R}{|}}{CH}-COOH \rightarrow \bigcirc\!\!-NH-\overset{\overset{\displaystyle S}{\|}}{C}-NH-\overset{\overset{\displaystyle R}{|}}{CH}-COOH$$

The derivatization of amino acids with PTC is the first step of the well known Edman degradation reaction. The PTC amino acid adducts are stable and easily separated by reversed phase HPLC technique. A single product is formed for each amino acid. Most reaction byproducts and all derivatization reagents are volatile, so they may be removed from the sample by vacuum drying.

Analysis of Fat and Water–soluble Vitamins[5]

The use of HPLC techniques for the analysis of vitamin Constituents has advantages over alternative assay methods. The traditional methods have relied upon different biological or chemical techniques for each vitamin. These methods are not only relatively costly for routine basis but also subject to poor selectivity and accuracy caused by interfering species in the sample. HPLC is advantageous for vitamin analysis since the separation eliminates interfering substances and several vitamin compounds are measured simultaneously.

The QA 1 Analyzer is capable of generating rapid and reproducible separations and quantitation for selected groups of vitamins in multivitamin formulations. Chromatographic conditions have been developed for both fat and water solube vitamins which utilize the same column so that only the mobile phase and detector wavelength need to be changed to convert from one method to the other. Sample preparation is one of the most important criteria prior to chromatographic analysis.

Sample Preparation for Fat–Soluble Vitamins

- ○ Grind 3 tablets; transfer to 40 ml caped tube
- ○ Solubilize in 10 ml DMSO/1% (w.v) Ammonium 1 Pyrrolidine Dithicarbamate
- ○ Heat 60 min at 60°C with occasional shaking; cool
- ○ Add 5 ml hexane; Vortex
- ○ Shake 30 min at ambient temperature
- ○ Centrifuge to separate phases
- ○ Remove 1 ml aliquots of hexane layer

○ Dry under N_2 stream

○ Reconstitute with 1 ml 2 Propanol

Analysis Conditions

○ Injection Volume : 10 µl
○ Column : Radial Pak C 18, (5 µm, 8mm × 10cm)
○ Mobile Phase : $CH_3CN/THF/H_2O$, (55 : 378)
○ Flow Rate : 4.0 ml/min
○ Flow Volume : 40 ml
○ Wavelength : 280 nm
○ Attenuation : 2 ↑ 5

Sample Preparation for Water–soluble Vitamins

○ Grind 1 tablet; transfer to 40 ml capped tube
○ Solubilize in 20ml DMSO/1% (w/v) Citric Acid
○ Heat 45 min at 60°C with occasional shaking; cool
○ Centrifuge
○ Inject supernatant

Analysis Conditions

○ Injection Volume : 10 µl
○ Column : Radial Pak C 18, (5 µm, 8mm × 10cm)
○ Mobile Phase : $CH_3CN/THF/H_2O$, (55 : 378)
○ Flow Rate : 4.0ml/min
○ Flow Volume : 40 ml
○ Wavelength : 280 nm
○ Attenuation : 2 ↑ 4

Determination of Drugs in Biological Matrices Using SPE Cartridges[6]

Using the Solid phase Extraction (SPE) with silica C18 cartridges for the sample preparation shows some limitations. The most common problem is coming from the sorbent drying effect of the cartridge during the preparation process, which leads to poor reproducibility or low compounds recovery. Another limitation is the strong retention of basic compounds due to silanol interaction between the silica and the positive charge of the base. Finally, most of the polar anlaytes are not retained on the cartridge due to the sorbent C18 group.

We can overcome all these problems by using Oasis HLB sorbent (Waters, USA) rather than using traditional, phases for SPE. The Oasis HLB (Hydrophilic Lipophilic Balance) sorbent is a macroporous copolymer made from a balanced ratio of two monomers, the lipophilic divinylbenzene that provides reversed phase property for analyte retention and the hydrophilic N vinylpyrolidone that allows sorbent to run dry without loss of recovery and reproducibility. The easiest way to use Oasis HLB cartridge is to apply the "One Dimension SPE method" as follows:

Condition the cartridge	→	Equilibrate with 1 ml water	→	Load 1 ml Sample	→	Wash with 1 ml 5% Methanol in Water

Evaporate & Reconstitute the Sample At 40°C with 200 µl Mobile Phase	←	Elute the Sample with 1 ml Methanol

One General SPE Method of a Wide Range of Compounds

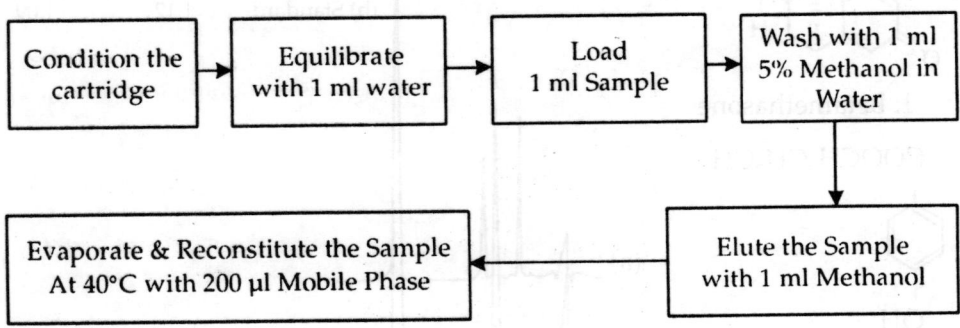

Acids

Sulfadiazine   Sulfamerazine   Sulfathiazole

Neutrals

Prednisolone   Betamethasone   Betamethasone valerate

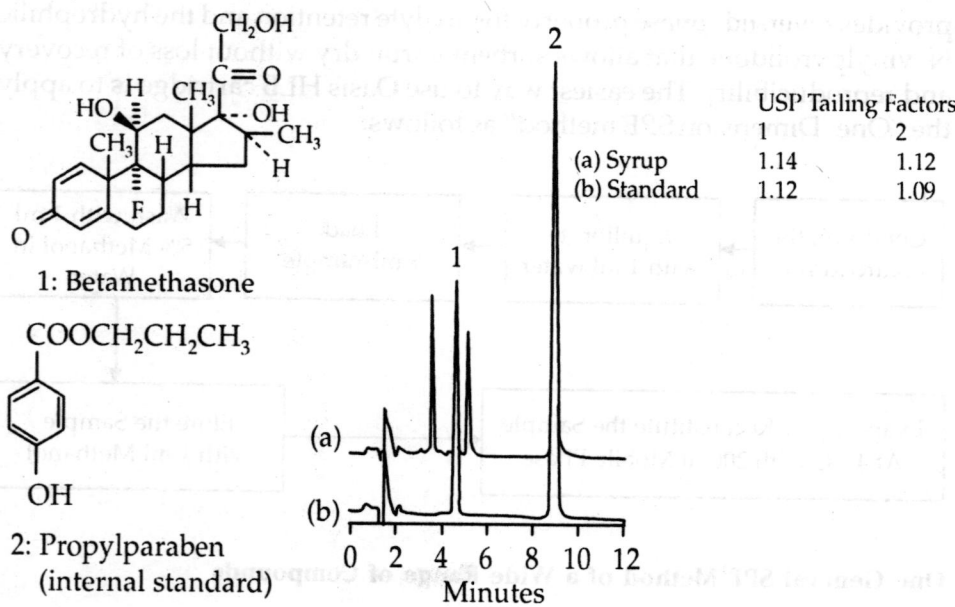

Base

Salbutamol

Bamethan

GLUCOCORTICOID : BETAMETHASONE
Standard and Syrup

1: Betamethasone

2: Propylparaben
(internal standard)

	USP Tailing Factors	
	1	2
(a) Syrup	1.14	1.12
(b) Standard	1.12	1.09

The "one dimension method" represents an excellent starting point for a wide range of compounds. It is a fast and easy protocol to obtain high recovery (> 85%) and consistent results (< 5% RSD). We can compare the percentage recovery and percentage RSD of Monocycline and Tetracycline using Oasis HLB cartridges and C 18 cartridges respectively under the same chromatographic conditions as follows:

○ Column   :   Symmetry Shield RP 8 (5 μm, 150 × 3.0 mm),

○ Mobile Phase   :   0.1 % TFA in water : acetonitrile : Methanol (19 : 7 : 2)

○ Detection   :   UV at 270 nm

○ Flow Rate   :   0.9 ml/min.

○ Injection volume :   20 μl.

Compounds	Concentration	Oasis HLB Cartridges		C18 Cartridges	
	µg/ml	Recovery (%)	RSD (%) n = 6	Recovery (%)	RSD (%) N = 6
Monocycline	2.5	94.8	1.40	40.7	0.82
Tetracycline	2.5	104	0.55	67.4	0.44

It is important to condition reversed phase silica based SPE cartridges properly before loading the sample. The conditioning solvent (typically methanol or acetonitrile) acts as a wetting agent and plays a key role by fully solvating the hydracarbon chains on the sorbent surface. Once the surface is wetted, water can displace this solvent, resulting in a sorbent surface that is in intimate contact with the water phase. Without the conditioning step, the aqueous sample cannot penetrate a reversed phase silica based sorbent's pores, where most of the analyte retention occurs. Improperly conditioned cartridges, which have been allowed to dry out, do not provide the same retention as cartridges that remain wetted. This leads to reduced recoveries with higher analytical variability.

APPLICATIONS

1. Standard Mixture of Organic Acids

			Peak identification
Column:	300 × 6.5 mm Chrompack organic Acids.	1.	Oxalic acid
Mobile:	0.01 N H_2SO_4 in water	2.	Cis Aconitic acid
Flow rate:	0.8 ml/min	3.	Oxaloacetic acid
Pressure:	1400 psi	4.	Pyruvic acid
Temperature:	35°C	5.	Tartaric acid
Detector:	UV, λ AT 210.	6.	Malic acid
Injection: Volume:	10 µl	7.	Lactic acid
Total run time:	15 minutes	8.	Formic acid
		9.	Propionic acid
		10.	Fumaric acid

Courtesy: Chrompack Chromatography notes

2. Vitamins: Tocopherol in Margarine

			Peak identification
Column:	Inertsil 5 Si (150 × 4.6 mm Chromsep Stainless Steel) Or, 150 × 4.6 mm conventional stainless steel	1.	α Tocopherol
		2.	β Tocopherol

Mobile Phase:	0.3% ethanol in n hexane	3. γ Tocopherol
Flow rate:	1 ml/min	4. δ Tocopherol
Temperature:	Ambient	
Detector:	Fluorescence, λ_{ex} = 300 nm, λ_{em} = 330 nm	
Injection: Volume::	20 µl	
Run time:	25 minutes	

3. Sweetners, Preservatives and Food Additives

Food industry uses preservatives (bonzoic acid or sorbic acid), sweetners (saccharin or aspartame) and additives (caffeine) in processed foods. Common uses of these exogenous ingredients have created a need for specific quality control of processed foods. Quantitatively the ingredients in processed food can be measured by HPLC as follows:

		Conc. In mixed standard (µg/ml)
Column:	Novapak C 18 (Waters USA) 150 × 4.6 mm, 5 µm	Saccharin : 300
Flow rate:	2 ml/min	Caffeine : 200
Mobile Phase:	CH_3CN : 0.5% Ammonium phosphate with 2% glacial acetic acid (15 : 85 (v/v))	Aspartame : 4000 Benzoic acid : 300
Temperature:	Ambient	Sorbic acid : 10
Detector:	UV, λ at 254 nm @ 0.1 AUFS	
Injection: Volume:	20 µl.	
Sample:	Standard	
Run time:	10 min.	

4. Qualitative and Quantitative Analysis of Catechines in Green Tea[7]:

Several recent laboratory studies have provided significant evidence supporting the role of tea and tea polyphenols (catechins) in the inhibition of cancer in animal models. The six major tea catechins are known to display biological activity are (+)-catechin (C), (–)-epicatechin (EC). (–)-epigallocatechin (EGC), (–) gallocatechin gallate (GCG), and (–)-epicatechin gallate (ECG). These natural products have strong antioxidant activity and have been shown to exhibit numerous potentially beneficial medicinal properties including inhibition of carcinogenesis, tumorogenesis and mutagenesis as well as the inhibition of tumour growth and metastasis[8]. In addition, these bioflavonoids have antibacterial and antiallergic properties[9].

Preparation of Catechin Standards

A standard aqueous solution containing 0.05 µg/µl of each of the six catechins and caffeine (as internal standard) was prepared.

Preparation of Green Tea Samples

A prcisely known amount of green tea leaves was steeped at 80°C for 10 min in 20 ml of water containing a known amount of caffeine as internal standard. The samples are then filtered through a 0.45 µm nylon filter and analysed directly by HPLC.

Chromatographic Conditions

Column	:	Symmetry C 18 (Waters, USA) (25 cm × 4.6 cm)
Mobile phase	:	Buffer A (Water + 0.05% TFA)
		Buffer B (60 : 40 MeOH CAN + 0.5% TFA)
Elution Mode	:	Gradient (0.5 min 10% B, 5 15 5 50 min 40% B)
Flow rate	:	1 ml/min.
Detector	:	PDA at 210 nm
Temperature	:	Ambient
Injection volume	:	210 µl.

5. Analysis of Steroid

Glucocorticoids have been analysed taking standards with different concentrations and surprisingly it was found that the retention times for all the standards are reproducible.

Chromatographic Conditions

Column	:	Symmetry C 18 or Novapak C 18 (15 cm × 3.9 cm)
Mobile Phase	:	Acetonitrile : Water (50 : 50)
Mode of elution	:	Isocratic
Flow rate	:	1 ml/mine
Temperature	:	30°
Detector	:	PDA at 210 nm
Injection Volume	:	210 µl.
Run Time	:	10 min.
Standard Mixture:		

GLUCOCORTICOIDS

Vo:Uracil

1: Prednisolone

2: Betamethasone

3: Prednisolone Acetate

4: Betamethasone Valerate

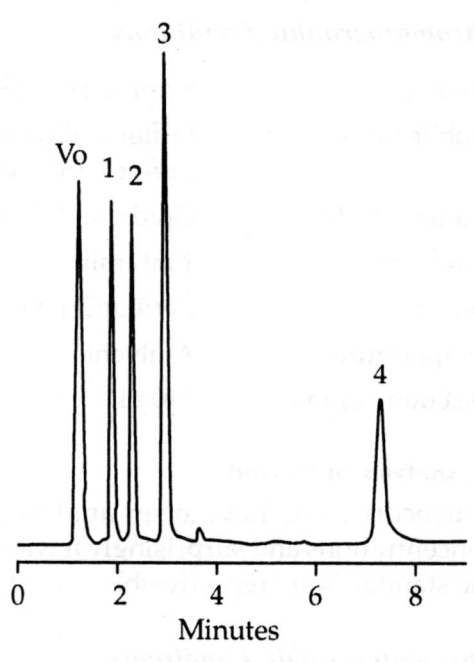

USP Tailing Factors
1:      1.1
2:      1.2
3:      1.1
4:      1.3

REFERENCES

1. Johnson, I. S. (1983). *Science*, **219**: 632.
2. Herring, S. (1982). Genetic Engineering News, (Sept./Oct.).
3. Water's Chromatography notes.
4. Dey, S. (2002). *Science and Culture*, **68**(1 4): 59-68.
5. Water's chromatography notes.
6. Waters chromatography notes.
7. Dalluge, J. J. and Bryant, C. *et. al.* (1998). of Chromatogr, A 793: 265-274.
8. Jankun, J., *et. al.*, (1997). *Nature*, 561.
9. Sakanaka, S., *et. al.*, (1989). *Agric Biol. Chem.*, **53**: 2301 2311.

SYSTEMATIC CLINICAL AND TOXICOLOGICAL ANALYSIS USING SOLID PHASE EXTRACTION

Vandana Dixit and Vyas M. Dixit*

ABSTRACT

This paper describes the principle and application of Solid Phase Extraction from biological matrices for detection of drugs and pharmaceuticals. Solid Phase Extraction processes can be divided in two parts. First sample preparation and second column extraction for isolation of the analyte. Depending upon the nature of matrix, sample preparation method may vary. Commonly used sample preparation methods for urine, serum/plasma samples are dilution and pH adjustment. For blood samples sonication, dilution and pH adjustment is the best choice. For tissues sample preparation is either protein precipitation or enzymatic digestion or direct blending of the tissue with solid support. To achieve sample preparation using SPE one should know the principles of SPE to get acceptable results. Several SPE methods for isolation and detection of drugs are reported and summarized. New SPE products with methodology and automation are also addressed here.

INTRODUCTION

Solid Phase Extraction (SPE) Technology has emerged as a powerful tool for sample preparation and chemical isolation. Since past 20-25 years this technology is being used for isolation and purification of different analytes. From small scale sample preparation to industrial scale chemical isolation this technology is being used in many areas such as pharmaceutical, clinical, technology is being used in many areas such as pharmaceutical, clinical, toxicological, environmental, biotechnology, water monitoring system, etc.

In systematic clinical and toxicological analysis major task is to detect and identify unknown compounds in a given matrix. The isolation and detection of drugs can be classified by two steps, the preparation of sample and the analysis of the drugs. Sample preparation of the matrix containing

*Anal Chem Pvt. Ltd, H-20/22 Ganga Darshan ADA Colony, Mehdauri, Allahabad 211 004, Tel: 0532-2545527, 2445264.

analyte is required for most analytical techniques such as TLC, HPLC, LC-MS, GC, GC-MS. A survey around the world indicates that more than 90% scientists recognize sample preparation as being "very important" or "moderately important"[1].

Traditional method for sample preparation is Liquid-Liquid extraction technique. In this method drugs are extracted from biological samples using immiscible solvent with several manipulations, combines extracts are then concentrated and reconstituted for analysis. Many problems associated with liquid-liquid extraction such as emulsion formation, interfering peaks, technique dependency cause to give variable results. More recent technique is SPE technique where prepared or diluted samples are directly loaded on the SPE column, after rinse the impurities are removed and compounds of interest are eluted in small amount of solvent. This gives clean extracts, little or no evaporation is required and there is no loss of analytes and therefore one gets reproducible results.

Today many types of SPE materials are commercially available[2]. In order to develop SPE procedure for biological samples, optimization of each step of procedure is very necessary. Factors that may affect the behavior of the relevant drugs during the extraction process include the selection of the suitable sorbent, pH of the sample, the clean-up step, the properties and the volume of the elution solvent, and the flow rate of the sample and elution solvent passing through the column. This paper presents the potentials of SPE for isolation and detection of drugs from biological matrices.

BIOLOGICAL SAMPLE PREPARATION

No matter what kind of extraction process is used for the analysis sample preparation of bioligical samples is the first important step in clinical and toxicological analysis. The main purposes of the sample preparation processes are listed below:

1. The detachment of the drugs from biological matrices.
2. Dilution and adjustment of pH to provide ionic strength and concentration for optimum extraction.
3. Removal of the lipophilic materials (proteins) and particulate matter which may interfere with analysis.

Sample Preparation for Biological Liquids

Biological liquids used for the analysis of drugs are urine, blood, and serum/plasma. In SPE technology plasma/serum can be treated simply by diluting matrix with suitable buffer solutions such as phosphate buffers. Table 1 shows the sample preparation methods applied in SPE for biological liquids.

TABLE 1: SAMPLE PREPARATION METHOD ON BIOLOGICAL SAMPLES USING SPE

Matrix	Sample Volume Initial/Final (mL)	Method	Reference
Plasma	2/8	Dilution	3
Plasma	½	Dilution	4
Plasma	1	Precipitation	5
Plasma	1	No Preparation	6
Plasma	1/10	Dilution	7
Serum	0.5	pH adjustment	8
Serum	½	Dilution	9
Serum	1	No Preparation	10
Urine	2/8	Dilution	3
Urine	2/9	Dilution	11
Urine	½	Dilution	4
Urine	10/12.5	Hydrolysis	12
Urine	3	Hydrolysis	13
Urine	1/1.5	Dilution	14
Urine	1/10	Dilution	7
Urine	5/7	Dilution	15
Urine	2	Hydrolysis	16
Blood	3/8	Dilution	17
Blood	1/7	Sonication/Dilution	18
Blood	2/12	Dilution	19
Blood	1/1.5	Dilution, Centri.	20
Blood	1/1	Sonication	21
Blood	1/20	Dilution	7

In case of whole blood and plasma/serum samples protein precipitation is a common method to obtain samples free of protein. This can be achieved by adding acids, salts, metallic ions, and organic solvents. Table 2 shows various types of precipitation methods.

Urine samples are generally diluted like plasma samples[3]. Blood samples can be diluted with buffer or organic solvent ans sonicated. General screening of the whole blood is reported by Chen *et al.*[18] using SPE column. The blood sample is first sonicated for the release of the drug and then diluted with phosphate buffer for adjustment of pH. Protein precipitation with $ZnSO_4$/ MeOH, acetonitrile, methanol is not suitable for sample preparation of whole blood in drug screening[22].

Sample Preparation of Tissue Samples

Extraction of drugs from tissue is most difficult task for forensic toxicologists. The most common method used in past for sample preparation in tissue were Stas-Otto method, the tungstate method, the ammonium sulfate method, the acid digestion method and the direct solvent extraction method. The advantages and disadvantages of these methods have been addressed by Jackson[23]. In 1970's, the enzymatic degistation technique was introduced[24]. The most common enzyme is substilisin-A which was reported by Osselton et al.[25-27] In 1980's Shankar et al.[28-29] reported that papain was suitable enzyme in obtaining the best recoveries. Most recently Matrix Solid Phase Dispersion (MSPD) extraction technology was introduced[30-31] where the tissue specimens are grinded with suitable adsorbent and loaded onto the same type of the column. This provides the high recoveries of the drugs with least amount of manipulation.

TABLE 2: VARIOUS PROTEIN PRECIPITATION METHODS[a]

Reagent	pH of Supernatant	Volume needed (mL)
Trchloroacetic, 10% (w/v)	1.4-2.0	0.2
Perchloric acid, 6% (wv)	< 1.5	0.4
Metaphosphoric acid, 5%	1.6-2.7	0.6
Tungstic acid	2.2-3.9	0.6
Methanol	8.5-9.5	2.0
Acetonitrile	8.5-9.5	1.5
Acetone	9-10	1.5
Ethanol	9-10	2.0
Ammonium sulphate (saturated)	7-0-7.7	2.0
CuSO4-Sodium tungstate	5.7-7.3	1.5
ZnSO4-NaOH	6.5-7.5	2.0
ZnSO4-BaOH	6.6-8.3	2.0

[a]Data taken from *J. Chromatogr.*, **226**: 445, 1981 (3)

Adjustment of pH for Ionic Strength

Like liquid/liquid extraction, dilution and adjustment of pH of the sample is an important factor in SPE also and can play a major role in the final results. The pH values of the sample and the extraction processes are dependent on the properties of the drugs and the interaction of the sorbent with the relevant drugs. For example octadecyl-bonded silica (C-18) is a non-polar sorbent. The main interaction is Van der Waals interactionsor hydrophobic interactions. Therefore, the sample should be diluted and pH of the sample should be adjusted in such a way that relevant drugs are in the uncharged forms. In another example, Drugtest I having multiple interactions such as non polar, ion exchange (sulphonic acid group) and polar (silanol groups) interactions together on silica support provides a wide range of properties for the sample manipulations. The basic drugs having

Pka greater than 8.0 in a given matrix can be diluted and adjusted to pH 6.0. At this pH the drugs and the sorbent (Drugtest I) both will be attached together by both by eletrostatic interactions andn hydrophobic interactions, and the impurities can be removed easily. By changing the pH and adding organic solvent drugs will be eluted. Total ionic strength of the sample plays an important role in Drugtest I. In general, a high concentration of species that can act as counter ions reduces the possibility of retention of ionic drugs. Therefore, a low ionic strength of the sample, often obtained by diluting the sample with a buffer solution, is advisable.

EXTRACTION OF DRUGS FROM BIOLOGICAL SAMPLES USING SOLID PHASE EXTRACTION TECHNOLOGY

A method of identifying narcotic analgesics in human urine using SPE technology was first reported in 1970 by Fujimoto *et al.*[32]. Amberlite XAD2 resins manufactured by Rohm and Hass was used as a solid support for sample preparation. US Varian as Bond Elut and Waters as Sep Pak introduced the smaller cartridges for sample preparation during 1975[33]. Since then,SPE has become greatly accepted technology in clinical, forensic toxicological laboratories[33]. Traditional method for sample preparation, liquid/liquid extraction has many problems, such as interfering peaks in the analysis, use of large amount of solvent, emulsion formation, non reproducible results and time consuming process. In SPE method higher selectivity, cleaner extracts, reduced solvents, removal emulsion formation, more reproducible results, higher throughput by means of automation[35-36] gives the end users more productivity.

The Principles of Solid Phase Extraction

Solid Phase Extraction Technology utilizes the principles of selective retention of analytes that characterizes the powerful seperation technique of HPLC. It is a physical extraction process that involves a liquid phase and a solid phase. The solid support (chemically modified silica surface/sorbent) has a greater attraction for the isolate (analyte) than the solvent in which the isolate is dissolved.

By choosing a proper solid support, packed in a polypropylene tube with open barrel configuration as shown in the figure, very selective extraction of high purity isolate can be achieved.

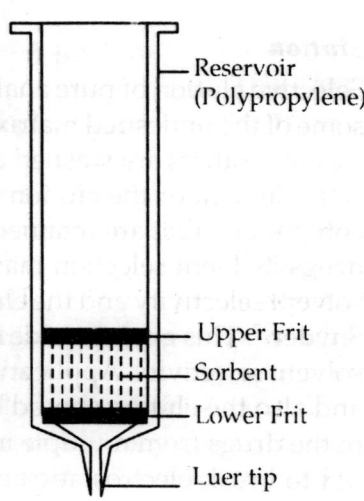
Reservoir (Polypropylene)
Upper Frit
Sorbent
Lower Frit
Luer tip

There are four steps involved in SPE process:

STEP I	:	Conditioning
STEP II	:	Application
STEP III	:	Rinse
STEP IV	:	Elution

Conditioning

Active sites of the support are not available to interact with analytes because the solid support is packed dry in a tube. Therefore conditioning the packed columns prior to sample application, to open the active sites of the support, is a key process in SPE technology to ensure reproducible retention of the analytes.

Application (Retention)

The compounds of interest (analytes or isolates, A) dispersed in a matrix containing other impurties (I) and undesired materials (U) are applied on to the column at a slow flow rate. A slow flow rate of sample application is necessary to achieve maximum retention of the analytes.

A	=	Analytes in matrix
I	=	Other matrix impurties
U	=	Undesired matrix constituents

Rinse

The column is rinsed with a specific solvent or combination of solvents to remove matrix impurities (I).

Elution

Selective elution of pure analytes (A) is achieved by using specific solvents, some of the undesired matrix constituents (U) are left behind on the support whereas others are washed out during rinse process.

The eluent or the elution solvent should be selective so that interfering compounds that are retained on the column should not be eluted with the drugs. Solvent selection may be achieved by considering the polarity, the solvent selectivity and the eluotropic strength which is greatly described by Snyder[37]. This gives a guide line to distinguish the solvent and strength of a solvent selectivity. Application of the sample on the column should be slow and also the elution should be slow to achieve better recovery. The elution of the drugs from multiple interaction column is achieved by changing the pH to break electrostatic bonding between the drugs and the sorbent. A selection chart is summarized in Table 3. US Varian has published a Hand book[38] "Sorbent Extraction" which provides useful information on SPE and its governing principles.

SAMPLE PREPARATION : FLOW DIAGRAM

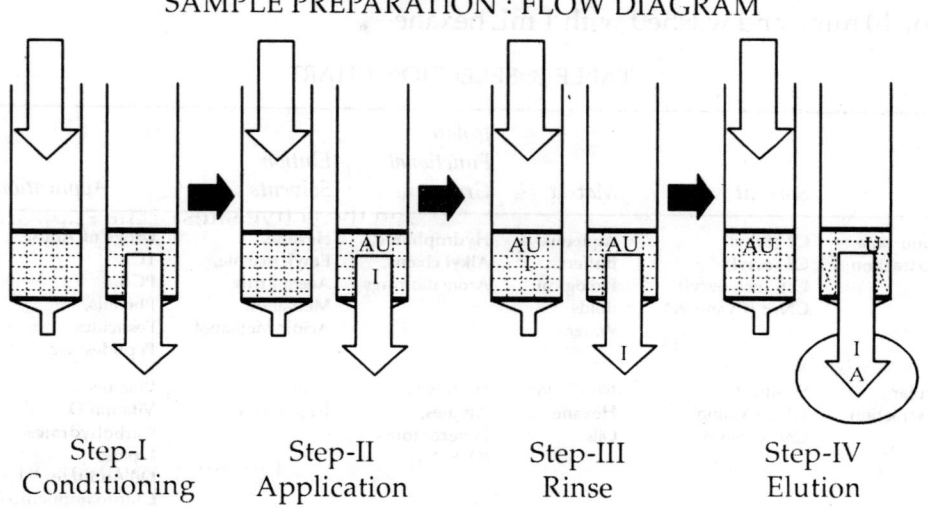

Step-I	Step-II	Step-III	Step-IV
Conditioning	Application	Rinse	Elution

Applications of SPE for Drug Screening

Extraction of broad range of drugs on single-mode column is very difficult. Therefore, multiplemode extraction columns were developed. Some examples are: Bond Elut Certify (US Varian), Clean Screen (World Wide Monitoring), Drugtest I and Drugtest II (Anal Chem Pvt Ltd, India).

Extraction of the drugs from tissue can be achieved by Solid-Matrix Dispersion method[30-31] but has received little attention so far[39]. Majority of publications have been reported for the extraction of individual drug or group of related drugs[17, 19, 12, 10, 40-44] using homogenization and enzymic digestion. Only a few publications on SPE applications for screening of wide variety of drug classes are reported[3, 14]. Of these one example is summarized below[14].

1. A Solid Phase Extraction Technique For Preparation of Drugs of abuse Samples from Urine. The extraction procedure for all classes of drugs of abuse from a single aliquot of urine begins with the addition of 5 mL of spiked urine, an internal standard (IS) and 2 mL of 100mM phosphate buffer (pH 6.0) to a large test tube. The specimen in the experiment was vortexed and the pH adjusted between 5-7. The Bond Elut Certify (a mixed mode) columns were connected to the Vacuum Manifold and conditioned with 2 mL of MeOH. Excess methanol was removed by washing with 2 mLof 100 mM phosphate buffer (pH 6.0). The Drug-spiked urine specimen was applied to the column and passed through the bed at a slow flow rate by applying

vacuum at approx. 2-3 in. Hg. One mL of 20 : 80 mixture of methanol and 100 mM phosphate buffer (pH 6.0) were transferred to the column. The sorbent bed was dried for 5 min under full vacuum (15 in. Hg.). The column was washed with 1 mL 1.0 M acetic acid solution, dried under full vacuum for 10 min., and washed with 1 mL hexane.

TABLE 3: SELECTION CHART

	Sorbent	Matrix	Isolate Functional Groups	Elution Solvents	Applications
Non polar Extraction	C2 (Ethyl) C8 (octyl) C18 (octadecyl) CNec (Cyano ec)	Aqueous: Buffers, Biological fluids, Water	Hydrophobic: Alkyl chains, Aromatic rings	Hexane, Ethyl Acetate, Acetonitrile, Methanol, Acidic Methanol	Drugs of Abuse, TCA, PCB, Phenols, Pesticides, Peptides, etc.
Polar Extraction	Si (silica) NH2 (Amino) CN (Cyano)	Non Polar: Hexane, Oils	Hydrophilic: Amines, Heteroatoms (O, S, N)	Acetone, Isopropanol,	Phenols, Vitamin D Carbohydrates, Lipids, Oil Additives, Chloroamphenicol, Beta Blockers, Cytochrome C, Trace Metals,
Cation Exchanger	ArCX (Benzene- sulfonic Acid)	Aqueous: Acidic buffers, Biological fluids, Water	Amines	Alkaline buffers, High Ionic Strength buffers	Pharmaceuticals, Aminocaproic acid, Catecholamines, Chlorophyll, Amino Acids, Tetracycline Gentamicin
Anion Exchanger	NH2 (Amino) QSAX (Quat)	Aqueous: Basic buffers, Biological fluids, Water	Carboxylic acids, Sulfonic acids, Phosphates	Acidic buffers, High Ionic Strength buffers	Vitamins, Organic Acids, Fatty Acids, Phosphates
Drugtest I	Multiple Interactions	Aqueous: Acidic buffers, Biological fluids, Water	Pharmaceutical, Cationic Drugs of Abuse	Strong Acids, Strong Bases, Organic Mixtures with Acids/Bases	Basic Drugs, Neutral Drugs

Elution of acidic drugs (barbiturates, phenytoin, methaqualone, etc.) was accomplished by passing a 4 mL aliquot of methylene chloride through the column and collecting it in a labeled tubes. For gas chromatography-flame ionization detection (GC-FID) analysis, 150 uL of alphenal (200 ug/10 mL of methanol) was added to each extract and used as the internal standard. Solvent was evaporated under a slow stream of nitrogen at room temperature and reconstituted in 100 uL ethyl acetate for further analysis.

To achieve the elution of basic drugs, the same column was rinsed with 6 mL of methanol. The sorbent bed was dried under full vacuum for 2 min and clean labeled test tubes placed on to the vacuum manifold. The basic drugs were eluted by passing 2 mL of 2% ammonium hydroxide in ethyl acetate through the column at a slow flow rate. For GC-FID analysis, 100 uL of N,N-dimethylformamide and 20 µL of methoxyphenamine (IS, 15 mg/10 mL methanol) were added to each extract. Solvent was evaporated to approx. 100 uL under a slow stream of nitrogen and injected for further analysis. The recovery of the various drugs were found to be greater than 80%.

RATIONAL BEHIND SOLID PHASE EXTRACTION TECHNOLOGY

Knowing nature of the analyte or analytes it is important to develop new materials. As described, the multiple mode materials are suitable for drug screening. Several materials have been prepared. Polymeric materials such as Polysorb MP-3 is based on lightly sulfonated C18 styrene-divinyl benzene co-polymer [45]. Patel and co-worker[46] have compared this material with multiple-mode bonded silica material and have found to some extent more useful. Since polymeric material are stable at high and low pH as well as have high surface area. But there are problems with the polymeric material as they have tendency to swell or shrink in different solvent and thus limits its application in drug screening.

Chemically modified silica cartridges, AccuCat is a mixed-mode material which bears anionic, cationic and polar interaction, has been used for catecholamines and their acidic and basic metabolites[13] from human urine.

Empore disks were developed by 3M and US Varian. It is a chemically modified C8 and C18 silica gel (8 µm, 60, Å) and 90% is embedded in a Teflon web. These disks have been used in environmental area[47]. There are some limitations with these disks as they have tendency to clog with dirty matrix. Some other materials have also been reported for SPE such as alumina.

Automation of SPE

When comparing liquid/liquid extraction with SPE, one of the advantages of SPE is automation of the methods. Recently manual SPE methods have been automated for the extraction of drugs. Various automated SPE systems that are made commercially available include AASP (VSPP), ASPEC (Gilson, WI), MilliLab (Bedford, MA), Zymate (Zymark, MA), Auto. Speed (Applied Seperation)[44, 48]. Automated procedure provides satisfactory recoveries of drugs with better or at least comparable reproducibility to manual SPE methods. It is advisable that to develop an automated method one should develop manual method first and transfer manual method to an automated method. The methods reported on automated systems have been more developed for single or limited drugs.

CONCLUSION

The use of SPE in sample preparation for biological matrices is a growing field. A multiple interaction solid phase extraction medium, a laboratory automation system using GC-MS and LC-MS aid in meeting the growing need for drug analysis. More attention has been given for the analysis of single drugs or a group of the drugs. Automation of SPE will improve efficiency and throughput.

REFERENCES

1. Majors, R. E. (1991). An overview of sample preparation. *LC-GC Int.*, **4**: 10.
2. Platoff, G. E., Gere, J. A. (1991). Solid Phase Extraction of abused drugs from urine. *Forensic Sci. Rev.*, **3**: 117.
3. Chen, X. H., Franke, J. P., Wijsbeek, J. and de Zeeuw, R. A. (1992). A single column procedure on Bond Elut Certify for systematic toxicological analysis of drugs in plasma and urine. *J. Forensic Sci.* **37**: 61.
4. Hattori, H., Takashima, E., Iwata, M., Yamada, T. and Suzuki, O. (1990). Rapid isolation of eleven analytical psychopharmaceuticals with Sep-Pak C18 cartridges and their sensitive analysis by gas chromatography with a flame thermionic detector. *Japan J. Forensic Toxicol.*, **8**: 117.
5. Musch, G., Massart, D. L. (1988). Isolation of basic drugs from plasma using solid-phas extraction wit a cyanopropyl bonded phase. *J. Chromatogr.*, **432**: 209.
6. Sioufi, A., Richard, J., Mangoni, P. and Godbollon, J. (1991). Determination of diclofenca in plasma using a fully automated analytical system combining liquid-solid extraction with liquid chromatography. *J. Chromatogr.*, **565**: 401.
7. Suzoki, O., Seno, H., Kumazawa, T. (1988). Rapid isolation of benzodiazapines with Sep-Pak C18 cartridges. *J. Forensic Sci.*, **33**: 1249.
8. Good, T. J., Andrews, J. S. (1981). The use of bonded phase extraction for rapid sample preparation of benzodiazepines and metabolites from serum for HPLC analysis. *J. Chromatogr. Sci.*, **19**: 562.
9. Mazhar, M. and Binder, S. R. (1989). Analysis of benzodiazzpines and tricyclic antidepressants in serum using a common solid phase clean-up and a common mobile phase. *J. Chromatogr.*, **497**: 201.
10. Roberts, G. M. and Hann, C. S. (1986). A rapid and reliable method for extraction and assay of TCA drugs in serum or plasma. *Biomed. Chromatogr.*, **1**: 49.
11. Elahi, N. (1980). Encapsulated XAD-2 extraction technique for a rapid extraction of drugs of abuse in urine. *J. Anal. Toxicol.*, **4**: 26.
12. Inoue, T., Suzuki, S. I. (1987). High-performance liquid chromatographic determination of triazolam and its metabolites in human urine. *J. Chromatogr.*, **4221**: 197.
13. Dixit, V. and Dixit, V. M. (1990). Sample preparation for the analysis of drugs of abuse samples. *Am. Clin. Lab.*, May/June: 46.
14. Logan, B. K., Stafford, D. T., Tebbett, I. R. and Moore, C. M. (1990). Rapid screening for 100 basic drugs and metabolites in urine using cation exchange solid-phase extraction and HPLC with diode array detection. *J. Anal. Toxicol.*, **14**: 154

15. Thompson, B. C., Kuzmack, J. M., I ηw, D. W. and Winslo, J. J. (1990). Copolymeric solid-phase extraction for quantitating drugs of abuse in urine by wide-bore capillary gas chromatography. *LC-GC Int.*, **3**: 55.

16. Dixit, V. and Dixit, V. M. (1990). A unique solid-phase extraction column for isolation of 11-nor- -9-tetrahydrocannabinol-9-carboxylic acid in human urine. *J. Liq. Chromatogr.*, **13**: 3313.

17. Anderson, W. H. and Fuller, D. C. (1987). A simplified procedure for the isolation, characterization, and identification of weak acid and neutral drugs from whole blood. *J. Anal. Toxicol.*, **11**: 198.

18. Chen, X. H., Frank, J. P., Wijsbeek, J., de Zeeuw, R. A. (1992). Isolation of acidic, neutral and basic drugs using a single mixed-mode solid-phase extraction column. *J. Anal .Toxicol.* **16**: 351.

19. Ford, B., Vine, J. and Watson, T. R. (1983). A rapid extractionmethod for acidic drugs in hemolyzed blood. *J. Anal. Toxicol.*, **7**: 116.

20. Leferink, J. G., Dankers, J. and Schotman, A. J. H. (1985). Doping analysis using solid-phase extraction and GC/MS with automated data handling; Proceedings of the 6th International Conference of Racing Analysts and Veterinarians; Hong Kong; p. 171.

21. Moore, C. M. and Tebbett, I. R. (1987). Rapid extraction of anti-inflammatory drugs in whole blood for HPLC analysis. *Forensic Sci. Int.*, **34**: 155.

22. Logan, B. K. and Stafford, D. T. (1990). A robust Solid-phase extraction method for basic drugs and metabolites in postmortem blood; Program-42nd Annual Meeting of American Academy of Forensic Sciences; Philadelphia, PA: Feb., p. 162.

23. Jackson, J. V. (1969). Extraction methods in toxicology. In: Clark EGC (ed.), *Isolation and Identification of Drugs*. The Pharmaceutical Press: London, UK; p. 22.

24. Jackson, J. V. (1986). Forensic Toxicology. In: Moffat, A. C., Jackson, J. A., Mos, M. S., Widoop, B. and Greenfield, E. S. (eds), *Clarke's Isolation and Identification of Drugs*, 2nd ed; The Pharmaceutical Press, London, UK; p. 44.

25. Osselton, M. D., Hammond, M. D. and Twitchett, P. J. (1977). The extraction and analysis of benzodiazapines in tissues by enzymic digestion and HPLC. *J. Pharm. Pharmac.*, **29**: 460.

26. Osselton, M. D. (1977). The release of basic drugs by enzymic digestion of tissues in cases of poisoning. *J. Forensic Sci. Soc.*, **17**: 189.

27. Osselton, M. D., Shaw, I. C. and Stevens, H. M. (1978). Enzymic digestion of liver tissue ro release barbiturates, salicylic acid and other acidic compounds in cases of human poisoning. *Analyst*, **103**: 1160.

28. Shankar, V., Damodaran, C. and Sekharan, P. C. (1987). Comparative evaluation of some enzymic digestion procedures in the release of basic drugs from tissue. *J. Anal. Toxicol.*, **11**: 164.

29. Shankar, V., Damodaran, C. and Sekharan, P. C. (1989). Barbiturate analysis in tissue by enzymic digestion and HPLC. *Forensic Sci. Int.*, **40**: 45.

30. Long, R. A., Soliman, M. M. and Steven, A. B. (1991). Matrix Solid Phase Dispersion (MSPD) extraction and gas Chromatographic screening of nine chlorinated pesticides in beef fat. *J. Assoc. Anal. Chem.*, **74**: 493.

31. Long, A. R., Crouch, M. D. and Barker, S. A. (1991). *J. Assoc. Anal. Chem.*, **74**: 667.

32. Fujimoto, J. M. and Wang, R. I. H. (1970). A method identifying narcotic analgesics in human urine after therapeutic doses. *Toxicol. Appl. Pharm.*, **16**: 186.

33. Majors, R. E. (1991). An overview of sample preparation. *LC-GC Int.*, **4**: 10.

34. McDowall, R. D. (1989) Sample preparation for biomedical analysis. *J. Chromatogram.*, **492**: 3.

35. Harkey, M. R. and Stolowitz, M. L. (1984). Solid-phase extraction techniques for bilogical specimens. In: Baselt, R. C. (ed.), *Advances in Analytical Toxicology*, Vol 1, Biomedical Publications: Foster City, CA; Chap 9.

36. Zief, M. and Kiser, R. (1988). Solid-phase extraction for sample preparation. J. T. Baker: Pghillipsburg, NJ.
37. Snyder, L. R. (1974). Clasification of the solvent properties of common liquids. *J. Chromatogr.*, **92**: 223.
38. Van Horn, K. C. (1985). Sorbent Extraction Technology: Analytichem International: Harbor City, CA.
39. Scheurer, J. and Moore, C. M. (1992). Solid-phase extraction of drugs from biological tissues-A review. *J. Anal. Toxicol.*, **16**: 264.
40. Boukhabza, A. Lugnier, A. A. J., Kintz, P. and Mangin, P. (1991). Simultaneous HPLC analysis of thehypnotic benzodiazapines nitrazepam, estazolam, flunitrazepam and trazolam in plasma. *J. Anal. Toxicol.*, **15**: 319.
41. Lloyd, J. B. F., Parry, D. A. (1989). Forensic applications of the determination of benzodiazapines in blood samples by micro column clean-up and HPLC with reductive mode electrochemical detection. *J. Anal. Toxicol.*, **13**: 163.
42. Matyska, M. and Golkiewicz, W. (1989). Quantitation of benzodiazipene hydrolysis products in urine using SPE and HPLC. *J. Liq. Chromatogr.*, **14**: 2796.
43. Narasimhachari, N. (1981). Evaluation of C18 Sep-Pak cartridges for biological sample clean-up for TCA assays. *J. Chromatogr.*, **225**: 189.
44. McDowall, R. D., Pearce, J. C. and Murkitt, G. S. (1986). Liquid-solid sample preparation in drug analysis. *J. Pharm. Biomed. Anal.*, **4**: 3.
45. Patel, R. M., Benson, J. R., Hometchko, D. and Marshall, G. (1990). Polymeric SPE of organic acids. *Int. Lab.* April: 38.
46. Patel, R. M., Jagodzinski, J. J., Benson, J. R. and Hometchko, D. (1990). Mixed-mode sorbent for sample preparation. *LC-GC Int.*, **3**: 49.
47. Markell, C., Hagen, D. F. and, Bunnelle, V. A. (1991). New Technologies in solid-phase extraction. *LC-GC Int.*, **4**: 10.
48. McDowall, R. D., Pearce, J. C. and Murkitt, G. S. (1989). Sample preparation using bonded silica; Recent experiences and new instrumentation. *TRAC*, **8**: 134.

BIOEQUIVALENCE OF GATIFLOXACIN BY HPLC METHOD—A CASE STUDY

U. Mandal*, M. Ganesan*, M. Jayakumar*, D. Senthil Rajan*, T. K. Pal*,
Mausumi Chakravarthi**, Arjita Roychowdhury**, Sangita Agarwal**
and T. K. Chattaraj**

ABSTRACT

Purpose: An efficient, simple and sensitive HPLC assay was developed for the determination of Gatifloxacin in human plasma sample to study bioequivalence of two Gatifloxacin tablets 400 mg (Gatifloxacin Tablets from SAGA Laboratories, Ahmedabad, India) as test formulation and GATILOX (BK 21135) from SUN Pharmaceuticals, Mumbai, India as a reference formulation in 12 healthy volunteers.

Methods: Gatifloxacin concentrations were analysed by reverse phase liquid chromatography and UV-detection ($\lambda = 290$ nm). The separation was achieved using Eurospher-100, C18 column (250 × 4.6 mm, 5 µ particle size) at room temperature. The Mobile phase consisted of a 50% phosphate buffer (4.76 gm KH_2PO_4 + 4.97 gm NaH_2PO_4 in 500 ml H_2O) and 50% Acetonitrile (ACN) volume by volume (v/v).

The study was conducted using a randomised 2-period cross over study with a washout period of 7 days. Plasma sample were obtained for a period of 0.5 -24 hrs. The bioequivalence between the two formulations was assessed by calculating individual peak plasma concentration (C_{max}) and area under the curve (AUC_{0-t}) ratios (test/reference). The confidence interval proposed was 0.8-1.25 as established by the US Food and drug administration agency.

Results: Gatifloxacin eluted at 2.5 min at a flow rate 1 ml/min. The mean absolute recovery of Gatifloxacin in plasma was 95.36% at 0.8 mcg/ml, 97.96% at 1.2 mcg/ml, 95.24% at 1.6 mcg/ml. The LOD (lower limit of detection) and LOQ (lower limit of Quantification) were found to be 0.2 mcg/ml and 0.25 mcg/ml respectively. The peak plasma levels of Gatifloxacin with both the preparations were achieved between, 1-2 hrs. The peak plasma

*Bioequivalence Study Centre, Department of Pharmaceutical Technology, Jadavpur University, Kolkata-700 032.
**N.R.S. Medical College and Hospital, A.J.C. Bose Road, Kolkata-700 014.

levels (C_{max}) of Gatifloxacin for the reference preparation Tablet Gatilox was ranged between 3.66-5.13 mcg/ml while test preparation was ranged between 3.55 -4.79 mcg/ml. On the basis of comparison of the AUC_{0-t} for Gatifloxacin after single dose administration the relative bioavailability of the test tablet Gatifloxacin 400 mg was 93.50% of that of reference preparation Gatilox.

Conclusion: The HPLC method adopted is simple, selective and suitable for bioequivalence study. Since 90% CI for both C_{max} and AUC_{0-t} lies within 0.8-1.25 confidence interval proposed by the Food and Drug administration it was concluded that Gatifloxacin 400 mg under test was bioequivalent to Gatilox 500 mg tablet in terms of both the rate and extent of absorption.

INTRODUCTION

Gatifloxacin is an advanced generation, 8-methoxyfluoroquinolone (Fig. 1). That is active against broad spectrum of pathogens including antibiotic resistant *Streptococcus pneumoniae*[1, 2]. Preliminary information indicates that gatifloxacin has an elimination half life of about 7-10 hrs. suggesting that once daily dosing will be appropriate for the treatment of susceptible pathogens. Development of a rapid, sensitive and selective method for the determination of gatifloxacin in human plasma is essential for understanding the pharmacokinetics of this drug when administered orally. Various assay procedures[3, 4] for the quantification of gatifloxacin in human plasma by LC-MS and microbial assay have been reported. But the objective of this work was to develop and validate an efficient simple and selective HPLC method with direct U-V detection in human plasma.

In this work the bioequivalence study of two gatifloxacin formulations (Test and reference) has been carried out by comparing the pharmacokinetic profiles of the drug.

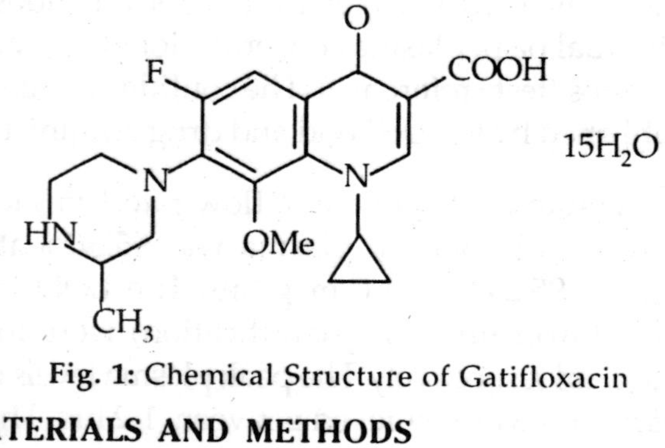

Fig. 1: Chemical Structure of Gatifloxacin

SUBJECTS, MATERIALS AND METHODS

Experimental

Twelve healthy male volunteers were studied aged 18-30 years (mean: 20.08 ± 3.9 years) and weight 48-69 kgs (mean 52.75 ± 6.48 kg). They were recruited from the panel of volunteers after excluding those with any evidence or history of relevant diseases of drug allergy or drug dependence. The subjects were informed about the nature of the compound they were going to take and informed consents in their mother tongue were signed by them.

Study Design

Prior to signing the consent form screening examination of the volunteers had been carried out which include complete physical and clinical examination of various biochemical and hematological tests.

With a view to study Bioequivalence of (Test preparation) of gatifloxacin 400 mg manufactured by SAGA LABORATORIES, INDIA (Ahmedabad) the subjects (12 Nos.) were given either Test or Reference preparation (GATILOX 400 mg) manufactured by SUN PHARMACEUTICAL INDIA LTD.) in two periods, randomised two-way complete cross-over design with a washout period of 7 days between two sessions. Each volunteer received all preparations (Test or Reference) and served as his own control.

Approval of this study was granted by DCGI, New Delhi (Drugs Controller General of India) and Institution Ethical Committee (IEC) of Jadavpur University, Kolkata.

Drug Administration

The tablets (Gatifloxacin 400 mg) were given orally in a single dose with 250 ml of water after a overnight fasting of at least 10 hrs.

Dietary Control

Standard breakfast lunch and dinner were served to the subjects at 3, 6-8 hrs. and 14 hrs. respectively after drug ingestion. Fluid intake has been controlled and no fluid except one cup of non-caffeine free soft drink was allowed till 3 hrs. post dose on the study day the volunteers were allowed normal activities TV watching excluding strenuous exercise.

Biological Samples

A total of 15 blood samples were collected from anticubal vein at 0 hr. (before drug administration) 0.5, 1, 1.5, 2, 3, 4, 6, 8, 10, 12, 18, 24, 36 and 48 hrs. in coded centrifuge tubes containing EDTA. Blood samples were centrifuged immediately, the plasma separated into duplicate polypropylene tubes and stored frozen at $-20^{\circ}C$. The tubes were labeled with volunteer code number, sampling time and study date.

Apparatus and Chromatographic Conditions

The instrument consisted of a HPLC, Knauer Germany (Model K2501) of isocratic system with a variable UV spectrophotometer set at 290 nm and an integrating software Eurochrom 2000. The mobile phase containing phosphate solution: Acetonitrile (phosphate solution: (ACN) = 50 : 50 v/v). The phosphate solution was prepared with 4.76 gm KH_2PO_4 + 4.97 gm NaH_2PO_4 in 500 ml H_2O. The sample was injected through a fixed loop Rheodyne injector system fitted with 20 ml Rhd. loop.

The column used was a Eurospher-100, C18, 250 × 4.6 mm, 5 μ particle size stainless steel.

Chemicals and Reagents

All salts and solvents were HPLC grade. Acetonitrile and water (HPLC grade) were from J.T. Baker, India whereas NaH_2PO_4 and KH_2PO_4, Methanol and Methylene chloride were from Merck, India.

Stock Solution

Stock solution of Gatifloxacin (8g/l) was prepared in double distilled water. Appropriate dilutions of the stock solutions were made before use.

Standard Solution

The working Gatifloxacin solution was perepared by diluting the stock solution (1 : 10) to a concentration of 0.8 gl^{-1}.

Calibration Curve

To obtain the calibration curve 100 μL of the working Gatifloxacin solution was diluted to 1 ml with blank serum. Aliquots of this solution were further diluted to obtain a series of solutions with concentrations of 0.25-8 μg ml^{-1} which were treated in an identical manner as described under extraction procedure. A 20 μl aliquot was injected and the mean drug peak area was plotted against the corresponding concentration (x). Each standard was replicated (n = 5). The linear regression equation obtained was as Y = 1.1797 − 0.02 (r = 0.9998).

Extraction Procedure

1 ml of plasma was taken in a stoppered test tube. To this 0.1 ml of dil H_3PO_4 was added and this mixture was sonicated for 1 minute. It was extracted with 4 ml of dichloromethane followed by vortexing for 1 minute and then centrifuged for 5 minutes with 4000 rpm. The organic layer was removed in a separate centrifuge tube with cap. 4 ml of the resulting organic layer was evaporated to dryness. The residue was reconstituted with 1 ml of mobile phase and the same was injected into HPLC.

Freeze Thaw Recovery

Plasma samples from volunteers were stored at –20°C ± 5°C. The pools of 0.25 (QCL), 0.75 (QCM) and 1.5 (QCH) mcg/ml of Gatifloxacin were prepared by addition of analyte to human blank plasma. These samples were analysed three times during the analysis period after taking out from the freezer and thawed.

Precision and Accuracy

Between - run precision and accuracy are determined from the low, medium and high QC (Quality Control) samples (QCL, QCM, QCH). A total of 5 replicates of each QC concentration were assayed on day 2 and 3. The QC samples concentrations were determined from three different calibration curves that were assayed with QC samples. Precision as expressed as % variation (% cv) while accuracy is measured as per cent nominal (% nominal). Within-run precision and accuracy are determined from a total of 5 replicates of each QC concentration. The low, medium and high QC samples (QCL, QCM, QCH) assayed on day 1. The QC samples concentration were determined from calibration curves. Precision is expressed as percent variation (% cv) and while the accuracy is measured as % nominal.

RESULTS

With the help of HPLC-UV method the quantification of Gatifloxacin was carried out and the drug appeared on chromatograph in approximately 2 to 2.5 minutes with no interferring peaks (Fig. 2).

Excellent linearity of drug concentration was observed over the range of 0.25 to 8.0 mcg/ml.

The lower Limit of Detection (LOD) and Lower Limit of Quantification (LOQ) were found to be 0.2 mcg/ml and 0.25 mcg/ml, respectively based on 1 ml of human plasma.

Between-run accuracy values (Table 1) (% nominal) were found to be > 95% for all the QC samples, while between run precision values (% cv) ranged from 1.87% to 4.73%. Within-run-precision values (% cv) (Table 2) did not exceed 10%. While the within-run accuracy values (% nominal) were > 95% for all the QC samples. Freeze Thaw recovery shown in Table 3 indicates that the sample were analysed three times during the analysis period and the samples were found to be stable.

The sensitivity of the assay was sufficient for determination of Gatifloxacin for a period of 1 to 24 hours.

The mean absolute recovery of Gatifloxacin was 95.36% at 0.8 mcg/ml, 97.96% at 1.2 mcg/ml and 95.24% at 1.6 mcg/ml.

Gatifloxacin (both reference and test) were well tolerated at the administered dose and no adverse effects were reported.

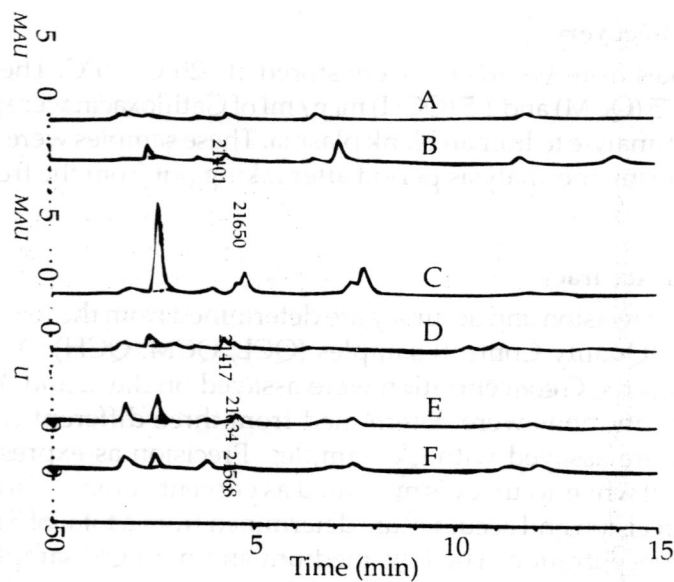

Fig. 2: Representative 15 min. chromatograph of Gatifloxacin

A—Blank Human Plasma, B—Human Plasma at 1.5 hrs., C—Human Plasma
at 2 hrs., D—Human Plasma at 4 hrs., E—Human Plasma at 8 hrs., F—Human
Plasma at 12 hrs., after a single oral dose of Gatifloxacin 400 mg tablet (Gatilox)

TABLE 1: BETWEEN-RUN PRECISION AND ACCURACY OF THE DETERMINATION
OF GATIFLOXACIN FROM SPIKED PLASMA SAMPLES (n = 13)

	QCL 0.4	QCM 0.8	QCH 2.5
Mean μg/ml	0.4070	0.7992	2.54
SD	0.0149	0.0152	0.1204
CV%	3.66	1.87	4.72
Absolute			
% bias	101.75	99.90	101.92

TABLE 2: WITHIN-RUN PRECISION AND ACCURACY OF THE DETERMINATION OF
GATIFLOXACIN FROM SPIKED PLASMA SAMPLES (n = 5)

	QCL 0.4	QCM 0.8	QCH 2.5
Mean mg/ml	0.3976	0.7964	2.513
SD	0.0116	0.0127	0.0902
CV%	2.93	1.601	3.58
Absolute			
bias %	99.40	99.55	100.55

TABLE 3: FREEZE THAW RECOVERY OF THE DETERMINATION OF GATIFLOXACIN
FROM SPIKED PLASMA SAMPLES (n = 3)

	QCL 0.25	QCM 0.75	QCH 1.5
Concentration mg/ml			
First cycle	0.248	0.705	1.43
Second cycle	0.234	0.729	1.41
Third cycle	0.239	0.743	1.46

Figure 3 shows the mean Gatifloxacin plasma concentration as a function of time after the oral administration of 400 mg Gatifloxacin of both brands (Standard and Test). The major pharmacokinetic parameters derived from the plasma concentration vs time on a two periods cross-over study are presented in Table 4.

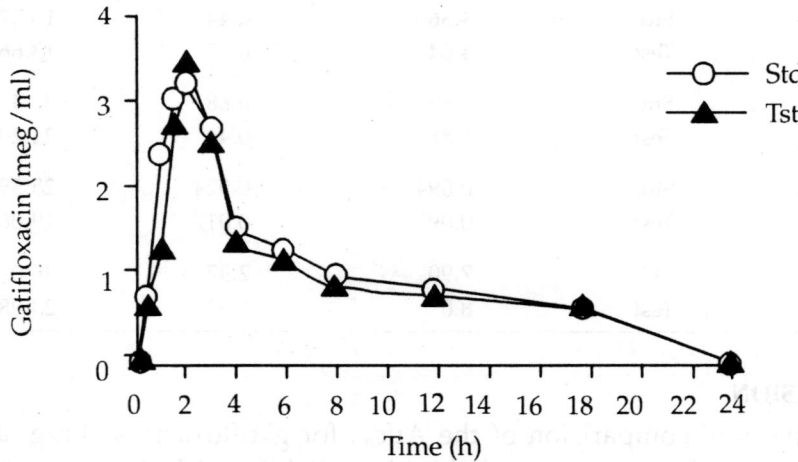

Fig. 3: Curves of the mean Plasma conc. vs. time (h) of gatifloxacin 400 mg oral dose

90% confidence interval (CI) for C_{max} lmc_{max}, Auc_{0-t} and $lnAuc_{0-t}$ values of test preparation of Tablet gatifloxacin were within the accepted limit of that of reference preparation (*i.e.* 0.8 → 1.2)] as proposed by DCGI, New Delhi.

DISCUSSION

This study of 12 healthy volunteers shows that a single oral dose of 400 mg of gaytifloxacin is well tolerated and is rapidly absorbed with mean T_{max} of 1.83 ± 0.44 hr and mean C_{max} of 4.04 ± 0.55 mg/ml.

As illustrated in Table 4 the mean values of T_{max}, C_{max} for both oral formulations were similar to those reported in the literature (3). Our results are in good agreement with earlier findings in term of T_{max} and C_{max} data.

We noted that Auc_{0-t} to be slightly greater at 33.68 µg.hr/ml while the earlier reports found the value to be 27.9 µg.h/ml. The earlier reports suggested a lower elimination half life from plasma of 6.8 h but our data suggested a slightly higher value than Stahlberg et al.[5].

TABLE 4: MEAN PHARMACOKINETIC PARAMETERS OBTAINED IN 12 HEALTHY VOLUNTEERS AFTER THE ADMINISTRATION OF BOTH 400 MG GATIFLOXACIN FORMULATIONS

		Mean	*SD*	*CV%*
AUC_{0-inf}	Std	33.68	4.31	12.78
mg/ml	Test	32.22	3.84	11.93
AUC_{0-t}	Std	25.26	2.91	11.54
mg/ml	Test	23.62	2.77	11.75
C_{max}	Std	4.366	0.44	10.07
mg/ml	Test	4.04	0.55	13.66
T_{max}	Std	1.79	0.68	38.4
(Hr)	Test	1.83	0.44	24.20
Kel/hr	Std	0.094	0.024	25.59
	Test	0.092	0.017	19.06
$t^{1/2}$	Std	7.90	2.37	30.01
(hr)	Test	8.0	1.92	23.98

CONCLUSION

On the basis of comparision of the Auc_{0-t} for gatifloxacin 400 mg, after single dose administration the relative bioavailability of Test preparation of tablet gatifloxacin was 93.50% of that of the reference preparation tablet Gatilox.

The validated HPLC method here proved to be simple, fast and reliable enough to be used in clinical pharmacokinetic studies of gatifloxacin in human.

The present study shows that gatifloxacin 400 mg Tablets was bioequivalent to Gatilox® tablet 400 mg.

ACKNOWLEDGEMENTS

The authors are thankful to SAGA LOBORATORIES, Ahmedabad, India for offering this job of Bioequivalence study. The Drugs Controller General of India (DCGI) is also thanked for the approval.

REFERENCES

1. Wise, R., Brenwald, N. P., Andrew, J. M. and Broswell, F. (1997). The activity of the methyl-piperazinyl fluoroquinolone CG5501: a comparision with other fluoroquivolones. *J. Antimicr Chemother*, **36**: 447-52.

2. Wakabayashi, E. and Mitsuhasi, S. (1994). *In vitro* activity of AM-1155, a novel 6-fluoro-8 methoxy qunolone. *Antimicr. Ag. Chemother.*, **38**: 594-601.

3. Wise, R., Andrew, J. M., Ashby, J. P. and Marshall, J. (1999). A study to determine the pharmaeokinetics and inflammatory fluid penetration of gatifloxacin following a single oral dose. *J. Antimicr Chemother.*, **44**: 701-704.

4. Vishwanathan, K., Bartlett, M. G. and Stewart, J. T. (2001). Determination of gatifloxacin in human plasma by liquid chromatography/electrospray tandem mass spectrometry. *Rapid Commun. Mass Spectrom.*, **15**(12): 915-9.

5. Stahlberg, H. J., Geohler, K. and Mignot, A. (1997). Multiple dose pharmacokinetics and exeretion balance of gatifloxacin, a new fluoroquinolone antibiotic, following oral administration of healthy caucasian volunteers. In Program and Abstracts of the Thirty-Seven Interscience Conference on Antimicrobiai Agents and Chemotherapy, Toronto, Canada, Abstract A71, 14. American Chemical Society for Microbiology, Washington DC.